NURSING:

SCOPE AND STANDARDS
OF PRACTICE

nurses
books
.org
The Publishing Program of ANA

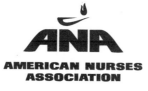

AMERICAN NURSES
ASSOCIATION

Washington, D.C.
2004

Library of Congress Cataloging-in-Publication Data

American Nurses Association.
  Nursing : scope and standards of practice / American Nurses Association.
    p. ; cm.
Includes bibliographical references and index.
  ISBN 1-55810-215-9 (alk. paper)
  1. Nursing—Standards—United States.
  [DNLM: 1. Nursing—standards. 2. Clinical Competence—standards.
WY16 A512n 2003] I. Title.

  RT85.5.A47 2003
  610.73'02'1873—dc22
                              2003020741

Disclaimer: The American Nurses Association (ANA) is a national professional association. This ANA publication—*Nursing: Scope and Standards of Practice*—reflects the thinking of the nursing profession on various issues and should be reviewed in conjunction with state board of nursing policies and practices. State law, rules, and regulations govern the practice of nursing, while *Nursing: Scope and Standards of Practice* guides nurses in the application of their professional skills and responsibilities.

Published by

nursesbooks.org
The Publishing Program of ANA

American Nurses Association
600 Maryland Avenue, SW
Suite 100 West
Washington, D.C. 20024-2571

1-800-274-4ANA

http://www.nursingworld.org

ISBN 1-55810-215-9

03SSNP   15M   12/03

Contributors

Work Group Members

Karen A. Ballard, MA, RN, Chairperson
Daria Arbogast, MSN, RN, CNP, OCN
Janet Boeckman, MSN, RN, CPNP
Patrick Conlon, MSN, RN-BC, CFNP, PNP-CS, CDE, BC-ADM, FAANP
Joyce A. Cox, MSN, RN, CNP, CRNFA
Nancy E. Dayhoff, EdD, RN, CNS
Jacqueline Fournier, MS, RN, CS
Linda Hozdic, MS, RN, CRNP, CNAA
Amy Murcko, MSN, APRN, CNAA,BC
Donna A. Peters, PhD, RN, FAAN
Gail A. Staudt, MSN, RNCS
Norma Stordahl, MSN, APRN,BC, CVN
Louise C. Waszak, PhD, CRNP

Congress of Nursing Practice and Economics

Anne M. Hammes, MS, RN, CNAA, Chairperson
Marva Wade, RN, Vice Chairperson

Members
Kathryn Ballou, PhD, RN
Joan M. Caley, MS, RN, CS, CNAA
Susan Foley Pierce, PhD, RN
Steven R. Pitkin, MN, RN
Lorna Samuels, MSN, ANP, GNP, RN, BC
Cathalene Teahan, MSN, RN, CNS
Susan Tullai-McGuinness, MPA, PhD, RN

Liaison members
Lola Fehr, MSN, RN, CAE, FAAN
Shirley Fields McCoy, MS, RN, C
Jeanne Surdo

ANA Staff
Department of Nursing Practice and Policy, American Nurses Association

Carol Bickford, PhD, RN,BC
Rita Munley Gallagher, PhD, RN,C
Mary Jean Schumann, MSN, RN, MBA CPNP
Yvonne Humes, MSA
Vernice Woodland

CONTENTS

PREFACE

The authority for the practice of nursing is based on a social contract that acknowledges the professional rights and responsibilities of nursing and includes mechanisms for public accountability. *Nursing's Social Policy Statement* (ANA, 2003) identifies that "nursing is the protection, promotion, and optimization of health and abilities, prevention of illness and injury, alleviation of suffering through the diagnosis and treatment of human response, and advocacy in the care of individuals, families, communities, and populations."

Nursing: Scope and Standards of Practice outlines the expectations of the professional role within which all registered nurses must practice. This scope statement and these updated standards of nursing practice guide, define, and direct professional nursing practice in all settings. *Nursing: Scope and Standards of Practice* is to be used in conjunction with *Nursing's Social Policy Statement* (ANA, 2003) and the *Code of Ethics for Nurses with Interpretive Statements* (ANA, 2001). These three resources provide a complete and definitive description for better understanding by specialty nursing organizations, policy makers, and the public of nursing practice and nursing's accountability to the public in the United States.

Development of Scope and Standards of Nursing Practice

The American Nurses Association (ANA) has actively engaged in scope of practice and standards development initiatives since the late 1960s. ANA published the first *Standards of Nursing Practice* for the nursing profession in 1973. The standards were generic in nature and focused on the basic nursing process—a critical thinking model applicable to all registered nurses—comprised of assessment, diagnosis, planning, implementation, and evaluation.

Over the years, specialty nursing organizations also have developed scope of practice statements and standards of practice for those registered nurses engaged in specialty practice, such as addictions, gerontology, pediatrics, hospice and palliative care, developmental disabilities, rehabilitation, psychiatric-mental health, oncology, nursing administration, informatics, professional development, and others. Some of these scopes and standards of practice were developed in collaboration with ANA; others were developed separately. Thus, the various scope and standards documents sometimes differed widely in purpose, scope, and format, and were limited in their ability to support an integrated picture of nursing and its contributions to health care.

In 1990, the ANA House of Delegates charged a task force to define the nature and purpose of standards of practice for nursing. The task force's report included a recommendation that the 1973 *Standards of Nursing Practice* be revised. A participative process was instituted that permitted incorporation of broad input and comments from state nurses associations and specialty nursing organizations.

In 1991, after a long and fruitful collaboration with specialty nursing organizations, ANA published *Standards of Clinical Nursing Practice (Clinical Standards)*. These professional clinical practice and performance standards established a common language and consistent format to clarify and strengthen nursing's ability to define the actual conduct of nursing practice within all practice areas. This initiative also established a framework within which specialty organizations and the ANA could work together to develop standards that foster a collaborative approach to decision-making concerning the practice of nursing. Throughout the 1990s, these standards significantly shaped nursing practice, served as a model for regulatory language, and provided a framework for other important works such as *Scope and Standards of Advanced Practice Registered Nursing* (ANA, 1996).

In 1995, the ANA Congress of Nursing Practice charged the Committee on Nursing Practice Standards and Guidelines with establishing a process for periodic review and revision, when necessary, of the standards documents. The process used in the development of the 1998 *Standards of Clinical Nursing Practice, 2nd Edition*, incorporated input from major stakeholders by:

(1) An assessment of the congruency of *Clinical Standards* with other contemporary ANA documents, e.g., *Nursing's Social Policy Statement* and the Code of Ethics;

(2) A survey of individual registered nurses as to their perceptions of the frequency of use and relevancy of *Clinical Standards* to their practice; and

(3) A survey of specialty nursing organizations as to the usefulness of *Clinical Standards* in regulatory and legislative activities.

Registered nurses throughout the country responded and affirmed the importance and usefulness of the original *Standards of Clinical Nursing Practice*.

In 2001, the Congress on Nursing Practice and Economics (CNPE) called for the establishment of a workgroup to conduct the review of *Standards of Clinical Nursing Practice, 2nd Edition*. The workgroup was assigned the task of incorporating into the new document the standards of practice for professional registered nurses, advanced practice registered nurses, and nurses in role specialties. Additional responsibilities included developing a corresponding contemporary statement of the scope of nursing practice.

The 2004 *Nursing: Scope and Standards of Practice* underwent a review process similar to the one implemented for the 1998 *Clinical Standards* with the significant addition of the opportunity for electronic web-based review that allowed individual comments. The CNPE workgroup:

- conducted an assessment for congruency of the new Scope and Standards with other ANA documents,

- distributed a working draft of the document to attendees of the 2002 ANA Convention,

- conducted a focus group at the 2002 ANA Convention,

- notified ANA's constituent member associations and the specialty nursing organizations that input was being requested on the draft document, and

- posted the draft document on ANA's www.NursingWorld.org web site for public review and comment by interested nurses and others.

All comments and suggestions were reviewed and considered by the workgroup in preparing this document. Reviews by the ANA Congress on Nursing Practice and Economics Committee on Clinical Practice Standards and Guidelines and the Congress on Nursing Practice and Economics culminated in the final edits of *Nursing: Scope and Standards of Practice*.

As with previous versions of this document, the real work begins now. The profession must incorporate the written word into practice settings across the country. The goal is to improve the health and well-being of all individuals, communities, and populations through the significant and visible contributions of registered nurses utilizing standards-based practice.

· · · · ·

Additional Content

To provide context for the development of Nursing: Scope and Standards of Practice (2004), the content of these appendices have been indexed:

- Appendix A: Timeline of the Development of Foundational Nursing Documents

- Appendix B: *Standards of Nursing Practice* (1973)

- Appendix C: *The Scope of Nursing Practice* (1987)

- Appendix D: *Standards of Clinical Nursing Practice* (1991)

- Appendix E: *Standards of Clinical Nursing Practice, 2nd Edition* (1998)

INTRODUCTION

Function of the Scope of Practice Statement

The scope of practice statement describes the *who, what, where, when, why,* and *how* of nursing practice. Each of these questions must be sufficiently answered to provide a complete picture of the practice and its boundaries and membership. The profession of nursing has one scope of practice that encompasses the full range of nursing practice. The depth and breadth in which individual registered nurses engage in the total scope of nursing practice is dependent upon education, experience, role, and the population served.

Function of Standards

Standards are authoritative statements by which the nursing profession describes the responsibilities for which its practitioners are accountable. Consequently, standards reflect the values and priorities of the profession. Standards provide direction for professional nursing practice and a framework for the evaluation of this practice. Written in measurable terms, standards also define the nursing profession's accountability to the public and the outcomes for which registered nurses are responsible.

Development of Standards

A professional nursing organization has a responsibility to its members and to the public it serves to develop standards of practice. Standards of professional nursing practice may pertain to general or specialty practice. As the professional organization for all registered nurses, the American Nurses Association (ANA) has assumed the responsibility for developing generic standards that apply to the practice of all professional nurses. Standards do, however, belong to the profession and, thus, require broad input into their development and revision. *Nursing: Scope and Standards of Practice* (*Scope and Standards*) describes a competent level of nursing practice and professional performance common to all registered nurses.

Assumptions

1. *A link exists between the professional work environment and the registered nurse's ability to practice.*

Nursing: Scope and Standards of Practice focuses primarily on the processes involved in the conduct of nursing practice and the performance of professional role activities. Although these standards apply to all registered nurses in all areas of practice, it is recognized that there is tremendous variability in these environments and practice settings. Recognizing the link between the professional work environment and the nurse's ability to practice, employers must provide an environment that supports nursing practice and decision-making.

2. *Nursing practice is individualized.*

The second assumption is that nursing practice is individualized to meet the unique needs of the patient or situation. This includes respect for the patient's and family's or support system's goals and preferences regarding care. Given that one of the registered nurse's primary responsibilities is education, nurses provide patients, colleagues, and others with appropriate information to make informed decisions regarding health care and healthcare issues, including health promotion, prevention of disease, and attainment of a dignified and peaceful death.

3. *Nurses establish partnerships.*

The third assumption is that the registered nurse establishes a partnership with the patient, family, support system, and other healthcare providers. In this partnership, the nurse works collaboratively to coordinate the care provided to the patient. The degree of participation by the patient, family, support system, and other healthcare providers will vary based upon needs, preferences, and abilities.

Organizing Principles

Nursing: Scope and Standards of Practice uses the term *patient* to include individuals, families, groups, communities, and populations to whom the registered nurse is providing services as sanctioned by the state nurse practice acts. The cultural, racial, and ethnic diversity of the patient must always be taken into account in providing nursing services.

Scope and Standards is generic in nature and applies to all professional registered nurses engaged in practice, regardless of clinical or functional specialty, practice setting, or educational preparation. When defining expectations associated with their particular area of specialty nursing practice, professional nursing organizations and groups may elect to develop more tailored and detailed scope of practice statements, standards, and associated measurement criteria built on the framework provided in *Nursing: Scope and Standards of Practice.*

The Standards of Nursing Practice content consists of Standards of Practice and Standards of Professional Performance, which include the following:

Standards of Practice

1 Assessment
2 Diagnosis
3 Outcomes Identification
4 Planning
5 Implementation
   5a Coordination of Care
   5b Health Teaching and Health Promotion
   5c Consultation
   5d Prescriptive Authority
6 Evaluation

Standards of Professional Practice

7 Quality of Practice
8 Education
9 Professional Practice Evaluation
10 Collegiality
11 Collaboration
12 Ethics
13 Research
14 Resource Utilization
15 Leadership

Standards of Practice

The six Standards of Practice describe a competent level of nursing care as demonstrated by the critical thinking model known as the nursing process. The nursing process includes the components of assessment, diagnosis, outcomes identification, planning, implementation, and evaluation. The nursing process encompasses all significant actions taken by registered nurses, and forms the foundation of the nurse's decision-making.

Several themes span all areas of nursing practice, are fundamental to many of the standards, and have emerged as being consistently and significantly influential in current nursing practice. These themes include:

- Providing age-appropriate and culturally and ethnically sensitive care
- Maintaining a safe environment
- Educating patients about healthy practices and treatment modalities
- Assuring continuity of care
- Coordinating the care across settings and among caregivers
- Managing information
- Communicating effectively
- Utilizing technology

These highlighted themes are reflected in the measurement criteria, although the wording may differ among the various standards. With future revisions of *Scope and Standards*, some of these themes may evolve into new standard statements.

Standards of Professional Performance

The nine Standards of Professional Performance describe a competent level of behavior in the professional role—including activities related to quality of practice, education, professional practice evaluation, collegiality, collaboration, ethics, research, resource utilization, and leadership. The last standard is new in this revision and addresses the leadership required of registered nurses in their practice. All registered nurses are expected to engage in professional role activities, including leadership, appropriate to their education and position. Registered nurses are accountable for their professional actions to themselves, their patients, their peers, and, ultimately, to society.

Measurement Criteria

Measurement criteria are key indicators of competent practice for each standard. *Nursing: Scope and Standards of Practice* includes criteria that allow the standards to be measured. For a standard to be met, all the listed measurement criteria must be met.

Standards should remain stable over time, as they reflect the philosophical values of the profession. Measurement criteria, however, can be revised more frequently to incorporate advancements in scientific knowledge and expectations for nursing practice. Additional measurement criteria that are applicable only to advanced practice registered nurses, or to those in nursing role specialties, are included for select standards of practice and professional performance.

In this document, words such as *appropriate* and *possible* are sometimes used. A document of this kind cannot account for all potential scenarios that the professional registered nurse might encounter in practice. The registered nurse will need to exercise judgment based on education and experience in determining what is appropriate or possible for a patient or in a particular situation. Further direction may be available from documents such as guidelines for practice or agency standards, policies, procedures, and protocols.

Relationship to Guidelines

Guidelines describe a process of patient care management, which has the potential for improving the quality of clinical and patient decision-making. As systematically developed statements based on available scientific evidence and expert opinion, practice guidelines address the care of specific patient populations or phenomena, whereas standards provide a broad framework for practice.

Summary

Nursing: Scope and Standards of Practice delineates the professional responsibilities of all professional registered nurses engaged in nursing practice, regardless of setting. *Scope and Standards* and available nursing practice guidelines can serve as a basis for:

- Quality improvement systems
- Data bases
- Regulatory systems
- Healthcare reimbursement and financing methodologies
- Development and evaluation of nursing service delivery systems and organizational structures
- Certification activities
- Position descriptions and performance appraisals
- Agency policies, procedures, and protocols
- Educational offerings

To best serve the public's health and the nursing profession, nursing must continue in its efforts to develop standards of practice and guidelines for practice. Nursing must also examine how standards and practice guidelines can be disseminated and used most effectively to enhance and promote the quality of practice. In addition, standards and practice guidelines must be evaluated on an ongoing basis, with revisions made as necessary. The dynamic nature of the healthcare environment and the growing body of nursing research provide both the impetus and the opportunity for nursing to ensure competent nursing practice in all settings for all patients and to promote ongoing professional development that enhances the quality of nursing practice.

SCOPE OF NURSING PRACTICE

Definition of Nursing

Nursing's Social Policy Statement, Second Edition (2003) builds on previous work and provides the following contemporary definition of nursing:

> *Nursing is the protection, promotion, and optimization of health and abilities, prevention of illness and injury, alleviation of suffering through the diagnosis and treatment of human response, and advocacy in the care of individuals, families, communities, and populations.*

This definition serves as the foundation for the following expanded content that describes the scope and standards of nursing practice.

Evolution of Nursing Practice

Contemporary nursing practice has its historical roots in the poorhouses, the battlefields, and the industrial revolutions in Europe and America. Initially nurses trained in hospital-based nursing schools and were employed mainly in private duty, providing care to patients in their homes. Florence Nightingale provided a foundation for nursing and the basis for autonomous nursing practice as distinctly different from medicine. Nightingale also is credited for identifying the importance of collecting empirical evidence, the underpinning of nursing's current emphasis on evidence-based practice, "What you want are facts, not opinions… The most important practical lesson that can be given to nurses is to teach them what to observe – how to observe – what symptoms indicate improvement – which are of none – which are the evidence of neglect – and what kind of neglect." (Nightingale, 1859, p. 105)

Although Nightingale recommended clinical nursing research in the mid 1800s, nurses did not follow her advice for more than 100 years. Nursing research was able to develop only as nurses received advanced educational preparation. In the early 1900s nurses received their advanced degrees in nursing education, which resulted in studies about nurses and nursing education. However, case studies on nursing interventions were conducted in the 1920s and 1930s, and the results published in the *American Journal of Nursing*.

Then in the 1950s, interest in nursing care studies began to arise. In 1952, the first issue of *Nursing Research* was published. In the 1960s, nursing studies began to explore theoretical and conceptual frameworks as a basis for practice. By the 1970s more doctorally prepared nurses were conducting research, and there was a shift to studies that focused on practice-related research and the improvement of patient care. By the 1980s there were more qualified nurse researchers than ever before, as well as an increasing availability of computers for collection and analysis of data. In 1985 the National Center for Nursing Research was established within the National Institutes of Health, putting nursing research into the mainstream of health research activities. (Grant and Massey, 1999)

In both World Wars, nurses responded to America's need for nurses to help care for the armed forces. In fact, by 1946, 31% of professional nurses had served with the troops. With advances in medical treatment and healthcare technology over the next sixty years, nurses in hospitals developed specialized nursing skills in both old and new areas of practice—medical–surgical nursing, pediatrics, anesthesia, midwifery, emergency care, mental health, critical care, neonatal care, and primary care. Nurses also increasingly engaged in addressing the need for public health interventions with at-risk communities and vulnerable populations; public health nursing was developed under its pioneer, Lillian Wald, at the Henry Street Settlement House in New York City.

During the last 50 years, nurse researchers (1950s) and nurse theorists (1960s and 1970s) greatly contributed to the expanding body of nursing knowledge with their studies of nursing practice and the development of nursing models and theories. These conceptual models and theories borrow from or share with other disciplines such as sociology, psychology, biology, and physics. For example, the work of Neuman and King built heavily on systems theory. There is also Levine's conservation model, Roger's science of unitary human beings, Roy's adaptation model, Orem's self-care model, Peplau's interpersonal relations model, and Watson's theory of caring. The 1980s brought revisions to these theories, as well as additional theories developed by nursing leaders, such as Johnson, Parse, and Leininger, that added to the theoretical thinking in nursing (George, 2002). In the 1990s, research studies tested and expanded these theories, which in turn continued to define and develop the discipline of nursing.

As nursing continued to evolve, four distinctly different advanced practice nursing groups developed to meet the increasingly complex needs of patients: clinical nurse specialist, nurse practitioner, certified nurse midwife, and certified registered nurse anesthetist. State laws and regulations have recognized and authorized the independent practice of nursing, encouraging greater numbers of registered nurses to pursue entrepreneurial activities, including establishing their own private practices. Similarly, the evolving healthcare delivery system has also provided exciting opportunities for registered nurses to move into other new roles.

Registered nurses throughout the decades have been social and political leaders and advocates, addressing many societal issues related to patient care, health, and wellness. Such issues have included protective labor laws, minimum wage, communicable disease programs, immunizations, well-baby/childcare, women's health, violence, reproductive health, end-of-life care, universal health care, social security, Medicare and Medicaid, the financing and reimbursement of health care, healthcare reform, ethics, mental health parity, confidentiality, workplace safety, and patients' rights.

Nursing has evolved into a profession with a distinct body of knowledge, university-based education, specialized practice, standards of practice, a social contract (*Nursing's Social Policy Statement,* 2003), and an ethical code (*Code of Ethics for Nurses with Interpretative Statements,* 2001). Registered nurses are concerned about the availability and accessibility of nursing care to patients, families, communities and populations. Registered nurses and the profession seek to ensure the integrity of nursing practice in all current and future healthcare systems.

The federal government collects data elements about the nursing workforce, the largest healthcare professional group in the U.S., as part of its numerous and disparate data collection activities. The most frequently cited consolidated source is the National Sample Survey of Registered Nurses (NSSRN), a sample survey of approximately 37,000 actively licensed registered nurses. The most recent National Sample Survey of Registered Nurses, conducted in March 2000 (U.S. HHS, 2002), identified that the estimated 2.7 million registered nurses are predominantly female and have an average age of 45.2 years. Increasing numbers of men are entering the profession and are estimated to number 147,000 or 5.4%. Hospitals, public/community health settings, ambulatory care settings and nursing homes/extended care continue to be the major employers of registered nurses. Although hospitals remain the primary employers, significant shifts to other settings are reflected by an increase since 1980 of 155% of registered nurses (RNs) employed in public health and community health settings and of 127% in ambulatory care settings. The number of registered nurses employed in nursing education has shown little change in the past two decades, despite a modest upward increase in the number of enrolled nursing students. A recent trend is the increased interest in nursing as a profession, prompting other professionals to change careers and enroll as second degree students in nursing education programs.

Integrating the Science and Art of Nursing

Nursing is a learned profession built upon a core body of knowledge reflective of its dual components of science and art. Nursing requires judgment and skill based upon principles of the biological, physical, behavioral, and social sciences. Nursing is a scientific discipline as well as a profession. Registered nurses employ critical thinking to integrate objective data with knowledge gained from an assessment of the subjective experiences of patients and groups. Registered nurses use this critical thinking process to apply the best available evidence and research data to the processes of diagnosis and treatment. Nurses continually evaluate quality and effectiveness of nursing practice and seek to optimize outcomes.

Nursing focuses on the promotion and maintenance of health and the prevention or resolution of disease, illness, or disability without restriction to a problem-focused orientation. The nursing needs of human beings are identified from a holistic perspective and are met within the context of a culturally sensitive, caring interpersonal relationship. Nursing includes the diagnosis and treatment of human responses to actual or potential health problems. Registered nurses employ practices that are restorative, supportive, and promotive in nature. *Restorative practices* modify the impact of illness or disease. *Supportive practices* are oriented toward modification of relationships or the environment to support health. *Promotive practices* mobilize healthy patterns of living, foster personal and family development, and support self-defined goals of individuals, families, communities, and populations.

Nursing is responsive to the changing needs of society and the expanding knowledge base of its theoretical and scientific domains. One of nursing's objectives is to achieve positive patient outcomes that maximize one's quality of life across the entire life-span. Registered nurses facilitate the interdisciplinary and comprehensive care provided by healthcare professionals, paraprofessionals, and volunteers. In other instances, nurses engage in consultation with other colleagues to inform decision-making and planning to meet patient care needs. Registered nurses often participate in interdisciplinary teams, where the overlapping skills complement each member's individual efforts.

All nursing practice, regardless of specialty, role, or setting, is fundamentally independent practice. Registered nurses are accountable for judgments made and actions taken in the course of their nursing practice. Therefore, the registered nurse is responsible for assessing individual competence and is committed to the process of lifelong learning. Registered nurses develop and maintain current knowledge and skills through formal and continuing education, and seek certification when available in their areas of practice. As independent practitioners, registered nurses are individually accountable for all aspects of their practice.

Registered nurses are bound by a professional code of ethics (*Code of Ethics for Nurses with Interpretive Statements*, 2001) and regulate themselves as individuals through peer review of practice. Peer review is a collegial process by which registered nurses are held accountable for practice. Peer evaluation fosters the refinement of knowledge, skills, and clinical decision-making at all levels and in all areas of clinical practice. Self-regulation by the profession of nursing assures quality of performance, which is the heart of the profession's social contract between the profession of nursing and society (*Nursing's Social Policy Statement*, 2003).

Registered nurses and members of various professions exchange knowledge and ideas about how to deliver high quality health care, resulting in overlaps and constantly changing professional practice boundaries. This multidisciplinary team collaboration among healthcare professionals involves recognition of the expertise of others within and outside one's profession and referral to those providers when appropriate. Such collaboration also involves some shared functions and a common focus on the same overall mission. By necessity, nursing's scope of practice has flexible boundaries.

Nursing practice is differentiated according to the registered nurse's educational preparation and level of practice, and is further defined by the role of the nurse and the work setting. Within each type of practice, individual nurses demonstrate competence along a continuum from novice to expert (Benner, 1982). Registered nurses can choose to develop expertise in a particular specialty and have this specialized knowledge base acknowledged through credentialing, such as certification or other mechanisms. Although advanced practice registered nurses continue to perform many of the same activities and interventions used by other nurses, the difference in their practice relates to a greater depth and breadth of knowledge, a greater degree of synthesis of data, and the increased complexity of skills and interventions.

Registered nurses regularly evaluate safety, effectiveness, and cost in the planning and delivery of nursing care. Nurses recognize that resources are limited and unequally distributed. As members of a profession, registered nurses work toward more equitable distribution and availability of healthcare services throughout the nation and the world.

The science of nursing is based on a critical thinking framework, known as the *nursing process,* composed of assessment, diagnosis, outcomes identification, planning, implementation, and evaluation. These steps serve as the foundation of clinical decision-making and are used to provide evidence-based practice. Wherever they practice, registered nurses use critical thinking to respond to the needs of the populations served, and use strategies that support optimal outcomes most appropriate to the patient or situation, being mindful of resource utilization.

Nursing is guided by standards of practice and standards of professional performance. *Standards* are authoritative statements by which the nursing profession describes the responsibilities for which its practitioners are accountable. Standards reflect the values and priorities of the profession and are based on research and knowledge from nursing and various other sciences and disciplines. Standards provide direction for professional nursing practice and a framework for the evaluation and improvement of practice. These ongoing assessments and evaluations are in keeping with nursing's commitment to lifelong learning, and to providing creative, deliberate, holistic, and up-to-date comprehensive care.

The art of nursing is based on a framework of caring and respect for human dignity. A compassionate approach to patient care carries a mandate to provide that care competently. Competent care is provided and accomplished through independent practice and collaborative partnerships. Collaboration may be with other colleagues or the individuals seeking support or assistance with their healthcare needs.

The art of nursing embraces dynamic processes that affect the human person including, for example, spirituality, healing, empathy, mutual respect, and compassion. These intangible aspects foster health. Nursing embraces healing. Healing is fostered by compassion, helping, listening, mentoring, coaching, teaching, exploring, being present, supporting, touching, intuition, empathy, service, cultural competence, tolerance, acceptance, nurturing, mutually creating, and conflict resolution.

The Professional Registered Nurse

A registered nurse (RN) is licensed and authorized by a state, commonwealth, or territory to practice nursing. Professional licensure of the healthcare professions was established to protect the public safety and authorize the practice of the profession. Requirements for authorization of nursing practice and the performance of certain professional nursing roles vary from jurisdiction to jurisdiction. The registered nurse's experience, education, knowledge, and abilities establish a level of competence.

The registered nurse is educationally prepared for competent practice at the beginning level upon graduation from an approved school of nursing (diploma, associate, baccalaureate, generic master's, or doctorate degree) and qualified by national examination for RN licensure. See Figure 1. Since 1965, the ANA has consistently affirmed the baccalaureate degree in nursing as the preferred educational preparation for entry into nursing practice.

Figure 1. Educational Path to Become a Registered Nurse

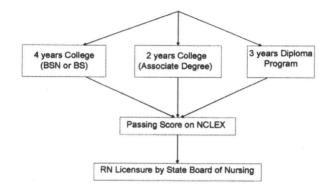

The registered nurse is educated in the art and science of nursing, with the goal of helping individuals and groups attain, maintain, and restore health whenever possible. Experienced nurses have become proficient in one or more practice areas or roles. These nurses may focus on patient care in clinical nursing practice specialties. Others function in roles that influence nursing and support the direct care rendered to patients by those professional nurses in clinical practice. Such specialized knowledge and experience may be acknowledged through an identified credentialing process. Credentialing organizations may mandate specific nursing educational requirements, as well as timely demonstrations of knowledge and experience in specialty practice.

Registered nurses may elect to pursue advanced academic studies to prepare for specialization in practice. Educational requirements vary by specialty and educational facility and may include completion of a national certification examination. See Figure 2. New models for educational preparation are evolving in response to the changing healthcare, education, and regulatory environments.

Figure 2. Professional Specialization for Registered Nurses

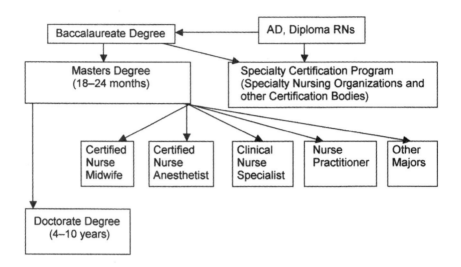

Advanced Practice Registered Nurses

Advanced practice registered nurses are RNs who have acquired advanced specialized clinical knowledge and skills to provide health care. These nurses are expected to hold a masters or doctorate degree. They build on the practice of registered nurses by demonstrating a greater depth and breadth of knowledge, a greater synthesis of data, increased complexity of skills and interventions, and significant role autonomy. As within all nursing practice, the level of expertise of the advanced practice registered nurse increases as they journey from novice to expert (Benner, 1982).

Advanced practice registered nurse (APRN) is the umbrella term used to identify the advanced practice roles of certified registered nurse anesthetist, certified nurse midwife, clinical nurse specialist, and nurse practitioner. Although the scope of practice for each of these advanced practice registered nurses is distinguishable from the others, there is an overlapping of knowledge and skills within these roles. The following descriptions are illustrative of these roles and not an exhaustive delineation of function.

Certified Registered Nurse Anesthetist: Certified registered nurse anesthetists (CRNAs) are graduates of nurse anesthesia educational programs accredited by the Council on Accreditation of Nurse Anesthesia Educational Programs or its predecessor, and have passed the certification examination administered by the Council on Certification of Nurse Anesthetists or its predecessor. CRNAs provide anesthesia and anesthesia-related care in the following domains: (1) the performance of pre-anesthetic preparation and evaluation; (2) anesthesia induction, maintenance, and emergence, including administration of appropriate drugs and techniques and local, regional, and general anesthesia, and the establishment of invasive monitoring; (3) post-anesthesia care; (4) acute and chronic pain management; and (5) associated clinical support functions, such as respiratory care and emergency resuscitation.

Certified Nurse-Midwife: Certified nurse-midwives (CNMs) are registered nurses, educated in the two disciplines of nursing and midwifery, who possess evidence of certification according to the requirements of the American College of Nurse-Midwives. Midwifery practice conducted by CNMs is the independent management of women's health care, including prescriptive authority. This practice focuses particularly on pregnancy, childbirth, the postpartum period, care of the newborn, and the family planning and gynecological needs of women. CNMs practice within a healthcare system that provides for consultation, collaborative management, or referral as indicated by the health status of the patient.

Clinical Nurse Specialist: Clinical nurse specialists (CNSs) are registered nurses, who have graduate level nursing preparation at the master's or doctoral level as a CNS. They are clinical experts in evidence-based nursing practice within a specialty area, treating and managing the health concerns of patients and populations. The CNS specialty may be focused on individuals, populations, settings, type of care, type of problem, or diagnostic systems subspecialty. CNSs practice autonomously and integrate knowledge of disease and medical treatments into the assessment, diagnosis, and treatment of patients' illnesses. These nurses design, implement, and evaluate both patient-specific and population-based programs of care. CNSs provide leadership in advancing the practice of nursing to achieve quality and cost-effective patient outcomes as well as provide leadership of multidisciplinary groups in designing and implementing innovative alternative solutions that address system problems and/or patient care issues. In many jurisdictions, CNSs, as direct care providers, perform comprehensive health assessments, develop differential diagnoses, and may have prescriptive authority. Prescriptive authority allows them to provide pharmacologic and nonpharmacologic treatments and order diagnostic and laboratory tests in addressing and managing specialty health problems of patients and populations. CNSs serve as patient advocates, consultants, and researchers in various settings.

Nurse Practitioner: Nurse practitioners (NPs) are registered nurses who have graduate level nursing preparation at the master's or doctoral level as a nurse practitioner. NPs perform comprehensive assessments and promote health and the prevention of illness and injury. These advanced practice registered nurses diagnose; develop differential diagnoses; order, conduct, supervise, and interpret diagnostic and laboratory tests; and prescribe pharmacologic and non-pharmacologic treatments in the direct management of acute and chronic illness and disease. Nurse practitioners provide health and medical care in primary, acute, and long-term care settings. NPs may specialize in areas such as family, geriatric, pediatric, primary, or acute care. Nurse practitioners practice autonomously and in collaboration with other healthcare professionals to treat and manage patients' health problems, and serve in various settings as researchers, consultants, and patient advocates for individuals, families, groups, and communities.

Registered Nurses in Role Specialties

As identified in *Nursing's Social Policy Statement, 2nd Edition* (2003), continuation of the profession is dependent on the education of nurses, appropriate organization of nursing services, continued expansion of nursing knowledge, and the development and adoption of policies. Such initiatives demand that registered nurses be adequately prepared for nursing role specialties, (those advanced levels of nursing practice that intersect with another body of knowledge), have a direct influence on nursing practice, and support the delivery of direct care rendered to patients by other registered nurses. Examples of nursing role specialty practice areas include administration, education, professional development, informatics, case management, quality initiatives, publishing, law, and research. Registered nurses in such role specialties generally hold master's or doctoral degrees. A registered nurse may enter a role specialty as a novice with goals to achieve the necessary education and experience for this type of advanced practice.

Settings for Nursing Practice

Nursing practice occurs whenever and wherever a registered nurse interacts with a patient, family, or group of persons, who experience or desire a change in their level of physical, mental, emotional, environmental, or spiritual well-being, or when the maintenance of their current level of well-being requires nursing action(s). The practice settings for the delivery of nursing care are continuously changing in response to the dynamic nature of today's healthcare environment. Settings may include, but are not limited to, academic medical centers, ambulatory health centers, clinics, communities, homes, hospices, hospitals, physician offices, and schools. In addition, nurses may practice in settings such as community nursing organizations, work sites, corporate offices, managed care organizations, correctional facilities, entrepreneurial private practices, pharmaceutical companies, professional nursing and healthcare organizations, and universities and colleges.

Registered nurses use telehealth technology in the delivery of nursing services in healthcare facilities, clinics, private offices, and the home. Nursing practice also occurs when nursing services are requested on behalf of a patient, such as a request for a consultation, or when registered nurses advocate for care that promotes health and prevents disease, illness, or disability for individuals or communities. Nurses through employment or voluntary participation, influence civic activities and the regulatory, and legislative arena at the local, state, national, or international level.

Continued Commitment to the Profession

Nursing is a dynamic profession, blending evidence-based practice with intuition, caring, and compassion to provide quality care. The nursing profession contracts with society to promote health, to do no harm, and to respond with skill and caring when change, birth, illness, disease, or death is experienced. Care is provided without regard to a person's background, identity, race, creed, circumstances, or religion.

Patients give nurses permission to enter their lives and share their most intimate life experiences. Registered nurses remain in nursing to promote, advocate for, and strive to protect the health, safety, and rights of those patients, families, communities, and populations. Registered nurses value their roles as advocates in dealing with barriers encountered in obtaining health care. Similarly, society values nursing care that resolves problems or manages health promoting behaviors (*Nursing's Social Policy Statement, 2003*).

Registered nurses experience rewarding challenges and opportunities in health care focusing on care of the whole person with various physical, psychological, and environmental needs and stressors. This involves commitment to help patients improve their physical and mental health, enrich their quality of life, reduce personal and environmental risks, and prevent disease, illness, and disability. Registered nurses prepare themselves to be resourceful, to respond to the challenges of delivering nursing care to individuals and communities, to incorporate technology into their art of caring, and to remain visionaries as the future unfolds.

Nursing also strives to strengthen individual practice through accountability and continued learning. Registered nurses seek to advance the profession through active involvement in civic activities, membership and support of professional associations, collective bargaining, and workplace advocacy. The registered nurse who articulates the goals, values, and integrity of nursing as described in *Code of Ethics for Nurses with Interpretive Statements* (ANA, 2001) ensures both nursing's commitment to the society it serves and the growth and progress of nursing itself. Registered nurses reflect these values in every day nursing practice through mentoring, listening, coaching, teaching, conflict resolution, and respecting diversity. The nurse owes the same duties to self as to others, including the responsibility to preserve professional integrity and safety, to maintain competence, and to continue personal and professional growth (ANA, 2001).

Nursing is an integral part of health care, and is indispensable to the functioning of the healthcare system. Registered nurses, as the largest group of healthcare professionals, utilize the power of their profession to make a positive impact on healthcare services and delivery. Nurses identify and champion the healthcare needs of the population, promote a safe environment, steward healthcare resources and promote universal access to healthcare services.

Professional Trends and Issues

Healthcare costs continue to escalate, prompting renewed calls for healthcare reform. Individuals and families face greater healthcare insurance premiums and deductibles as employers and insurance entities decrease their payment share for the same or, often lesser, coverage. Increasing numbers of uninsured persons join many of those with healthcare benefits in deferring preventive health and dental care and only seeking healthcare services for acute illness or injury. Self treatment and reliance on complementary and alternative therapies continue to garner an increasing market share as individuals become more involved in their own care and seek new ways to achieve health.

Today, as in the past, nursing remains pivotal to improving the health status of the public and ensuring safe, effective, quality care. Registered nurses provide a critical safety net in health care, but have been consistently invisible in the practice and reimbursement environments. Nursing care activities have not been identified by unique coding systems that would allow billing as direct services. Research continues to demonstrate and reaffirm that effective nursing care from registered nurses prevents adverse patient outcomes (Aiken et al, 2002). Although the evidence of nursing's contribution and its monetary value to health care is slowly being recognized, the current shortage of registered nurses compounds the issue and must be addressed from both the supply and demand perspectives.

The American Nurses Association and more than 100 specialty nursing organizations are identifying key initiatives and generating solutions to counter the nursing shortage, which is the major issue that needs to be addressed by the profession, healthcare industry, and government in the next decade (ANA, 2002). Nursing shortages have occurred cyclically throughout the last century. Unfortunately, the problems associated with an increasingly difficult healthcare work environment (control over the practice environment, staffing levels, mandatory overtime, salaries and benefits, availability of ancillary and technical supports, and access to staff development and education), as well as the burdensome structure of the healthcare system, have not been adequately addressed.

Currently, registered nurses and nurse faculty match the demographics of our aging population (National Sample Survey of Registered Nurses, March 2000; U.S. HHS, 2002). The adequate supply of registered nurses in clinical practice settings can only be replenished and supplemented if sufficient numbers of students enroll in nursing education programs that are supported with appropriate numbers of available teaching faculty. However, the nursing faculty shortage is projected to worsen in the next few years with the anticipated retirements of the aging faculty. Experienced registered nurses elect to remain in clinical settings or move to other healthcare venues, rather than suffer pay cuts associated with today's low faculty salaries. With faculty departing for retirement, a secondary consequence of significant magnitude will be a decline in research and publications so necessary for generating nursing knowledge.

Registered nurses must proactively deal with constant change and must be prepared for an evolving healthcare environment that includes advanced technologies. The incorporation of technologies, however, is not without risk, and demands due diligence by registered nurses to consider the impact on the scope of nursing practice and the ethical implications for healthcare consumers, as well as for the nurse.

The healthcare industry has been challenged to improve patient safety, both patient and practitioner satisfaction, patient outcomes, and the profitability of the healthcare organization (Kennedy, 2003). In 1999, the Institute of Medicine (IOM) described the nation's healthcare system as fractured, prone to errors, and detrimental to safe patient care (IOM, 1999). The IOM has identified six aims for improvement so that the healthcare system is: safe, effective, patient-centered, timely, efficient, and equitable (IOM, 2001).

In 2002, the American Nurses Association stated "if problems in the work environment are not addressed, nurses will not be able to sufficiently protect patients" (ANA, 2002). The impact of nursing staffing upon patient safety has been clearly demonstrated (Needleman & Buerhaus, 2003). The healthcare industry must address the adverse effects on nurses and patient safety of inadequate staffing, healthcare errors, episodes of failure to rescue, and the looming nursing shortage.

Nursing as a profession continues to address ongoing issues around entry into practice, the autonomy of advanced practice, continued competency, multistate licensure, and the appropriate educational credential for professional certification.

Registered nurses as lifelong learners must have available the appropriate and adequate professional development and continuing education opportunities to maintain and advance skills and enhance competencies. Such a positive climate promotes mentoring and speeds the transition of the registered nurse from novice to expert. Significant variation in employers' support for the professional development of nurse employees forces registered nurses to find innovative learning solutions, and may even prompt migration to another nursing environment that values and encourages the contributions of the lifelong learner.

Whatever the practice venue, in the next decade, registered nurses will continue to partner with others to seek to advance the nation's health through many initiatives, such as meeting the goals of Healthy People 2010 to increase the quality and years of healthy life and eliminate health disparities. Such partnerships truly reflect the definition of nursing and illustrate the essential features of contemporary nursing practice:

- Provision of a caring relationship that facilitates health and healing.

- Attention to the range of human experiences and responses to health, disease, and illness within the physical and social environments.

- Integration of objective data with knowledge gained from an appreciation of the patient's or group's subjective experience.

- Application of scientific knowledge to the processes of diagnosis and treatment through the use of judgment and critical thinking.

- Advancement of professional nursing knowledge through scholarly inquiry.

- Influence of social and public policy to promote social justice.
(*Nursing's Social Policy Statement*, 2003)

STANDARDS OF NURSING PRACTICE

STANDARDS OF PRACTICE

STANDARD 1. ASSESSMENT

The registered nurse collects comprehensive data pertinent to the patient's health or the situation.

Measurement Criteria:

The registered nurse:

Collects data in a systematic and ongoing process.

Involves the patient, family, other healthcare providers, and environment, as appropriate, in holistic data collection.

Prioritizes data collection activities based on the patient's immediate condition, or anticipated needs of the patient or situation.

Uses appropriate evidence-based assessment techniques and instruments in collecting pertinent data.

Uses analytical models and problem-solving tools.

Synthesizes available data, information, and knowledge relevant to the situation to identify patterns and variances.

Documents relevant data in a retrievable format.

Additional Measurement Criteria for the Advanced Practice Registered Nurse:

The advanced practice registered nurse initiates and interprets diagnostic tests and procedures relevant to the patient's current status.

STANDARD 2. DIAGNOSIS

The registered nurse analyzes the assessment data to determine the diagnoses or issues.

Measurement Criteria:

The registered nurse:

Derives the diagnoses or issues based on assessment data.

Validates the diagnoses or issues with the patient, family, and other healthcare providers when possible and appropriate.

Documents diagnoses or issues in a manner that facilitates the determination of the expected outcomes and plan.

Additional Measurement Criteria for the Advanced Practice Registered Nurse:

The advanced practice registered nurse:

Systematically compares and contrasts clinical findings with normal and abnormal variations and developmental events in formulating a differential diagnosis.

Utilizes complex data and information obtained during interview, examination, and diagnostic procedures in identifying diagnoses.

Assists staff in developing and maintaining competency in the diagnostic process.

STANDARD 3. OUTCOMES IDENTIFICATION

The registered nurse identifies expected outcomes for a plan individualized to the patient or the situation.

Measurement Criteria:

The registered nurse:

Involves the patient, family, and other healthcare providers in formulating expected outcomes when possible and appropriate.

Derives culturally appropriate expected outcomes from the diagnoses.

Considers associated risks, benefits, costs, current scientific evidence, and clinical expertise when formulating expected outcomes.

Defines expected outcomes in terms of the patient, patient values, ethical considerations, environment, or situation with such consideration as associated risks, benefits and costs, and current scientific evidence.

Includes a time estimate for attainment of expected outcomes.

Develops expected outcomes that provide direction for continuity of care.

Modifies expected outcomes based on changes in the status of the patient or evaluation of the situation.

Documents expected outcomes as measurable goals.

Additional Measurement Criteria for the Advanced Practice Registered Nurse:

The advanced practice registered nurse:

Identifies expected outcomes that incorporate scientific evidence and are achievable through implementation of evidence-based practices.

Identifies expected outcomes that incorporate cost and clinical effectiveness, patient satisfaction, and continuity and consistency among providers.

Supports the use of clinical guidelines linked to positive patient outcomes.

STANDARD 4. PLANNING

The registered nurse develops a plan that prescribes strategies and alternatives to attain expected outcomes.

Measurement Criteria:

The registered nurse:

Develops an individualized plan considering patient characteristics or the situation (e.g., age and culturally appropriate, environmentally sensitive).

Develops the plan in conjunction with the patient, family, and others, as appropriate.

Includes strategies within the plan that address each of the identified diagnoses or issues, which may include strategies for promotion and restoration of health and prevention of illness, injury, and disease.

Provides for continuity within the plan.

Incorporates an implementation pathway or timeline within the plan.

Establishes the plan priorities with the patient, family, and others as appropriate.

Utilizes the plan to provide direction to other members of the healthcare team.

Defines the plan to reflect current statutes, rules and regulations, and standards.

Integrates current trends and research affecting care in the planning process.

Considers the economic impact of the plan.

Uses standardized language or recognized terminology to document the plan.

Additional Measurement Criteria for the Advanced Practice Registered Nurse:

The advanced practice registered nurse:

Identifies assessment, diagnostic strategies, and therapeutic interventions within the plan that reflect current evidence, including data, research, literature, and expert clinical knowledge.

Selects or designs strategies to meet the multifaceted needs of complex patients.

Includes the synthesis of patients' values and beliefs regarding nursing and medical therapies within the plan.

Additional Measurement Criteria for the Nursing Role Specialty:

The registered nurse in a nursing role specialty:

Participates in the design and development of multidisciplinary and interdisciplinary processes to address the situation or issue.

Contributes to the development and continuous improvement of organizational systems that support the planning process.

Supports the integration of clinical, human, and financial resources to enhance and complete the decision-making processes.

STANDARD 5. IMPLEMENTATION

The registered nurse implements the identified plan.

Measurement Criteria:

The registered nurse:

Implements the plan in a safe and timely manner.

Documents implementation and any modifications, including changes or omissions, of the identified plan.

Utilizes evidence-based interventions and treatments specific to the diagnosis or problem.

Utilizes community resources and systems to implement the plan.

Collaborates with nursing colleagues and others to implement the plan.

Additional Measurement Criteria for the Advanced Practice Registered Nurse:

The advanced practice registered nurse:

Facilitates utilization of systems and community resources to implement the plan.

Supports collaboration with nursing colleagues and other disciplines to implement the plan.

Incorporates new knowledge and strategies to initiate change in nursing care practices if desired outcomes are not achieved.

Additional Measurement Criteria for the Nursing Role Specialty:

The registered nurse in a nursing role specialty:

Implements the plan using principles and concepts of project or systems management.

Fosters organizational systems that support implementation of the plan.

Standard 5a: Coordination of Care

The registered nurse coordinates care delivery.

Measurement Criteria:

The registered nurse:

Coordinates implementation of the plan.

Documents the coordination of the care.

Measurement Criteria for the Advanced Practice Registered Nurse:

The advanced practice registered nurse:

Provides leadership in the coordination of multidisciplinary health care for integrated delivery of patient care services.

Synthesizes data and information to prescribe necessary system and community support measures, including environmental modifications.

Coordinates system and community resources that enhance delivery of care across continuums.

STANDARD 5B: HEALTH TEACHING AND HEALTH PROMOTION

The registered nurse employs strategies to promote health and a safe environment.

Measurement Criteria:

The registered nurse:

Provides health teaching that addresses such topics as healthy lifestyles, risk-reducing behaviors, developmental needs, activities of daily living, and preventive self-care.

Uses health promotion and health teaching methods appropriate to the situation and the patient's developmental level, learning needs, readiness, ability to learn, language preference, and culture.

Seeks opportunities for feedback and evaluation of the effectiveness of the strategies used.

Additional Measurement Criteria for the Advanced Practice Registered Nurse:

The advanced practice registered nurse:

Synthesizes empirical evidence on risk behaviors, learning theories, behavioral change theories, motivational theories, epidemiology, and other related theories and frameworks when designing health information and patient education.

Designs health information and patient education appropriate to the patient's developmental level, learning needs, readiness to learn, and cultural values and beliefs.

Evaluates health information resources, such as the Internet, within the area of practice for accuracy, readability, and comprehensibility to help patients access quality health information.

STANDARD 5c: CONSULTATION

The advanced practice registered nurse and the nursing role specialist provide consultation to influence the identified plan, enhance the abilities of others, and effect change.

Measurement Criteria for the Advanced Practice Registered Nurse:

The advanced practice registered nurse:

Synthesizes clinical data, theoretical frameworks, and evidence when providing consultation.

Facilitates the effectiveness of a consultation by involving the patient in decision-making and negotiating role responsibilities.

Communicates consultation recommendations that facilitate change.

Measurement Criteria for the Nursing Role Specialty:

The registered nurse in a nursing role specialty:

Synthesizes data, information, theoretical frameworks and evidence when providing consultation.

Facilitates the effectiveness of a consultation by involving the stakeholders in the decision-making process.

Communicates consultation recommendations that influence the identified plan, facilitate understanding by involved stakeholders, enhance the work of others, and effect change.

STANDARD 5D: PRESCRIPTIVE AUTHORITY AND TREATMENT

The advanced practice registered nurse uses prescriptive authority, procedures, referrals, treatments, and therapies in accordance with state and federal laws and regulations.

Measurement Criteria for the Advanced Practice Registered Nurse:

The advanced practice registered nurse:

Prescribes evidence-based treatments, therapies, and procedures, considering the patient's comprehensive healthcare needs.

Prescribes pharmacologic agents based on a current knowledge of pharmacology and physiology.

Prescribes specific pharmacological agents and/or treatments based on clinical indicators, the patient's status and needs, and the results of diagnostic and laboratory tests.

Evaluates therapeutic and potential adverse effects of pharmacological and non-pharmacological treatments.

Provides patients with information about intended effects and potential adverse effects of proposed prescriptive therapies.

Provides information about costs, alternative treatments and procedures, as appropriate.

STANDARD 6. EVALUATION

The registered nurse evaluates progress toward attainment of outcomes.

Measurement Criteria:

The registered nurse:

Conducts a systematic, ongoing, and criterion-based evaluation of the outcomes in relation to the structures and processes prescribed by the plan and the indicated timeline.

Includes the patient and others involved in the care or situation in the evaluative process.

Evaluates the effectiveness of the planned strategies in relation to patient responses and the attainment of the expected outcomes.

Documents the results of the evaluation.

Uses ongoing assessment data to revise the diagnoses, outcomes, the plan, and the implementation as needed.

Disseminates the results to the patient and others involved in the care or situation, as appropriate, in accordance with state and federal laws and regulations.

Additional Measurement Criteria for the Advanced Practice Registered Nurse:

The advanced practice registered nurse:

Evaluates the accuracy of the diagnosis and effectiveness of the interventions in relationship to the patient's attainment of expected outcomes.

Synthesizes the results of the evaluation analyses to determine the impact of the plan on the affected patients, families, groups, communities, and institutions.

Uses the results of the evaluation analyses to make or recommend process or structural changes, including policy, procedure or protocol documentation, as appropriate.

Continued ▸

Additional Measurement Criteria for the Nursing Role Specialty:

The registered nurse in a nursing role specialty:

Uses the results of the evaluation analyses to make or recommend process or structural changes, including policy, procedure or protocol documentation, as appropriate.

Synthesizes the results of the evaluation analyses to determine the impact of the plan on the affected patients, families, groups, communities, and institutions, networks, and organizations.

STANDARDS OF PROFESSIONAL PERFORMANCE

STANDARD 7. QUALITY OF PRACTICE

The registered nurse systematically enhances the quality and effectiveness of nursing practice.

Measurement Criteria:

The registered nurse:

Demonstrates quality by documenting the application of the nursing process in a responsible, accountable, and ethical manner.

Uses the results of quality improvement activities to initiate changes in nursing practice and in the healthcare delivery system.

Uses creativity and innovation in nursing practice to improve care delivery.

Incorporates new knowledge to initiate changes in nursing practice if desired outcomes are not achieved.

Participates in quality improvement activities. Such activities may include:

Identifying aspects of practice important for quality monitoring.

Using indicators developed to monitor quality and effectiveness of nursing practice.

Collecting data to monitor quality and effectiveness of nursing practice.

Analyzing quality data to identify opportunities for improving nursing practice.

Formulating recommendations to improve nursing practice or outcomes.

Implementing activities to enhance the quality of nursing practice.

Developing, implementing, and evaluating policies, procedures, and/or guidelines to improve the quality of practice.

Participating on interdisciplinary teams to evaluate clinical care or health services.

Participating in efforts to minimize costs and unnecessary duplication.

Analyzing factors related to safety, satisfaction, effectiveness, and cost/benefit options.

Analyzing organizational systems for barriers.

Implementing processes to remove or decrease barriers within organizational systems.

Continued ▸

Additional Measurement Criteria for the Advanced Practice Registered Nurse:

The advanced practice registered nurse:

Obtains and maintains professional certification if available in the area of expertise.

Designs quality improvement initiatives.

Implements initiatives to evaluate the need for change.

Evaluates the practice environment and quality of nursing care rendered in relation to existing evidence, identifying opportunities for the generation and use of research.

Additional Measurement Criteria for the Nursing Role Specialty:

The registered nurse in a nursing role specialty:

Obtains and maintains professional certification if available in the area of expertise.

Designs quality improvement initiatives.

Implements initiatives to evaluate the need for change.

Evaluates the practice environment in relation to existing evidence, identifying opportunities for the generation and use of research.

STANDARD 8. EDUCATION

The registered nurse attains knowledge and competency that reflects current nursing practice.

Measurement Criteria:

The registered nurse:

Participates in ongoing educational activities related to appropriate knowledge bases and professional issues.

Demonstrates a commitment to lifelong learning through self-reflection and inquiry to identify learning needs.

Seeks experiences that reflect current practice in order to maintain skills and competence in clinical practice or role performance.

Acquires knowledge and skills appropriate to the specialty area, practice setting, role, or situation.

Maintains professional records that provide evidence of competency and life long learning.

Seeks experiences and formal and independent learning activities to maintain and develop clinical and professional skills and knowledge.

Additional Measurement Criteria for the Advanced Practice Registered Nurse:

The advanced practice registered nurse:

Uses current healthcare research findings and other evidence to expand clinical knowledge, enhance role performance, and increase knowledge of professional issues.

Additional Measurement Criteria for the Nursing Role Specialty:

The registered nurse in a nursing role specialty:

Uses current research findings and other evidence to expand knowledge, enhance role performance, and increase knowledge of professional issues.

STANDARD 9. PROFESSIONAL PRACTICE EVALUATION

The registered nurse evaluates one's own nursing practice in relation to professional practice standards and guidelines, relevant statutes, rules, and regulations.

Measurement Criteria:

The registered nurse's practice reflects the application of knowledge of current practice standards, guidelines, statutes, rules, and regulations.

The registered nurse:

Provides age appropriate care in a culturally and ethnically sensitive manner.

Engages in self-evaluation of practice on a regular basis, identifying areas of strength, as well as areas in which professional development would be beneficial.

Obtains informal feedback regarding one's own practice from patients, peers, professional colleagues, and others.

Participates in systematic peer review as appropriate.

Takes action to achieve goals identified during the evaluation process.

Provides rationales for practice beliefs, decisions, and actions as part of the informal and formal evaluation processes.

Additional Measurement Criteria for the Advanced Practice Registered Nurse:

The advanced practice registered nurse engages in a formal process, seeking feedback regarding one's own practice from patients, peers, professional colleagues, and others.

Additional Measurement Criteria for the Nursing Role Specialty:

The registered nurse in a nursing role specialty engages in a formal process seeking feedback regarding role performance from individuals, professional colleagues, representatives, and administrators of corporate entities, and others.

STANDARD 10. COLLEGIALITY

The registered nurse interacts with and contributes to the professional development of peers and colleagues.

Measurement Criteria:

The registered nurse:

Shares knowledge and skills with peers and colleagues as evidenced by such activities as patient care conferences or presentations at formal or informal meetings.

Provides peers with feedback regarding their practice and/or role performance.

Interacts with peers and colleagues to enhance one's own professional nursing practice and/or role performance.

Maintains compassionate and caring relationships with peers and colleagues.

Contributes to an environment that is conducive to the education of healthcare professionals.

Contributes to a supportive and healthy work environment.

Additional Measurement Criteria for the Advanced Practice Registered Nurse:

The advanced practice registered nurse:

Models expert practice to interdisciplinary team members and healthcare consumers.

Mentors other registered nurses and colleagues as appropriate.

Participates with interdisciplinary teams that contribute to role development and advanced nursing practice and health care.

Additional Measurement Criteria for the Nursing Role Specialty:

The registered nurse in a nursing role specialty:

Participates on multi-professional teams that contribute to role development and, directly or indirectly, advance nursing practice and health services.

Mentors other registered nurses and colleagues as appropriate.

STANDARD 11. COLLABORATION

The registered nurse collaborates with patient, family, and others in the conduct of nursing practice.

Measurement Criteria:

The registered nurse:

Communicates with patient, family, and healthcare providers regarding patient care and the nurse's role in the provision of that care.

Collaborates in creating a documented plan, focused on outcomes and decisions related to care and delivery of services, that indicates communication with patients, families, and others.

Partners with others to effect change and generate positive outcomes through knowledge of the patient or situation.

Documents referrals, including provisions for continuity of care.

Additional Measurement Criteria for the Advanced Practice Registered Nurse:

The advanced practice registered nurse:

Partners with other disciplines to enhance patient care through interdisciplinary activities, such as education, consultation, management, technological development, or research opportunities.

Facilitates an interdisciplinary process with other members of the healthcare team.

Documents plan of care communications, rationales for plan of care changes, and collaborative discussions to improve patient care.

Additional Measurement Criteria for Nursing Role Specialty:

The registered nurse in a nursing role specialty:

Partners with others to enhance health care and, ultimately, patient care through interdisciplinary activities, such as education, consultation, management, technological development, or research opportunities.

Documents plans, communications, rationales for plan changes, and collaborative discussions.

STANDARD 12. ETHICS

The registered nurse integrates ethical provisions in all areas of practice.

Measurement Criteria:

The registered nurse:

Uses the *Code of Ethics for Nurses with Interpretive Statements* (ANA, 2001) to guide practice.

Delivers care in a manner that preserves and protects patient autonomy, dignity, and rights.

Maintains patient confidentiality within legal and regulatory parameters.

Serves as a patient advocate assisting patients in developing skills for self advocacy.

Maintains a therapeutic and professional patient–nurse relationship with appropriate professional role boundaries.

Demonstrates a commitment to practicing self-care, managing stress, and connecting with self and others.

Contributes to resolving ethical issues of patients, colleagues, or systems as evidenced in such activities as participating on ethics committees.

Reports illegal, incompetent, or impaired practices.

Additional Measurement Criteria for the Advanced Practice Registered Nurse:

The advanced practice registered nurse:

Informs the patient of the risks, benefits, and outcomes of healthcare regimens.

Participates in interdisciplinary teams that address ethical risks, benefits, and outcomes.

Additional Measurement Criteria for the Nursing Role Specialty:

The registered nurse in a nursing role specialty:

Participates on multidisciplinary and interdisciplinary teams that address ethical risks, benefits, and outcomes.

Informs administrators or others of the risks, benefits, and outcomes of programs and decisions that affect healthcare delivery.

STANDARD 13. RESEARCH

The registered nurse integrates research findings into practice.

Measurement Criteria:

The registered nurse:

Utilizes the best available evidence, including research findings, to guide practice decisions.

Actively participates in research activities at various levels appropriate to the nurse's level of education and position. Such activities may include:

Identifying clinical problems specific to nursing research (patient care and nursing practice).

Participating in data collection (surveys, pilot projects, formal studies).

Participating in a formal committee or program.

Sharing research activities and/or findings with peers and others.

Conducting research.

Critically analyzing and interpreting research for application to practice.

Using research findings in the development of policies, procedures, and standards of practice in patient care.

Incorporating research as a basis for learning.

Additional Measurement Criteria for the Advanced Practice Registered Nurse:

The advanced practice registered nurse:

Contributes to nursing knowledge by conducting or synthesizing research that discovers, examines, and evaluates knowledge, theories, criteria, and creative approaches to improve healthcare practice.

Formally disseminates research findings through activities, such as presentations, publications, consultation, and journal clubs.

Additional Measurement Criteria for the Nursing Role Specialty:

The registered nurse in a nursing role specialty:

Contributes to nursing knowledge by conducting or synthesizing research that discovers, examines, and evaluates knowledge, theories, criteria, and creative approaches to improve health care.

Formally disseminates research findings through activities, such as presentations, publications, consultation, and journal clubs.

STANDARD 14. RESOURCE UTILIZATION

The registered nurse considers factors related to safety, effectiveness, cost, and impact on practice in the planning and delivery of nursing services.

Measurement Criteria:

The registered nurse:

Evaluates factors such as safety, effectiveness, availability, cost and benefits, efficiencies, and impact on practice when choosing practice options that would result in the same expected outcome.

Assists the patient and family in identifying and securing appropriate and available services to address health-related needs.

Assigns or delegates tasks based on the needs and condition of the patient, potential for harm, stability of the patient's condition, complexity of the task, and predictability of the outcome.

Assists the patient and family in becoming informed consumers about the options, costs, risks, and benefits of treatment and care.

Additional Measurement Criteria for the Advanced Practice Registered Nurse:

The advanced practice registered nurse:

Utilizes organizational and community resources to formulate multidisciplinary or interdisciplinary plans of care.

Develops innovative solutions for patient care problems that address effective resource utilization and maintenance of quality.

Develops evaluation strategies to demonstrate cost effectiveness, cost benefit, and efficiency factors associated with nursing practice.

Additional Measurement Criteria for the Nursing Role Specialty:

The registered nurse in a nursing role specialty:

Develops innovative solutions and applies strategies to obtain appropriate resources for nursing initiatives.

Secures organizational resources to ensure a work environment conducive to completing the identified plan and outcomes.

Develops evaluation methods to measure safety and effectiveness for interventions and outcomes.

Promotes activities that assist others, as appropriate, in becoming informed about costs, risks, and benefits of care, or of the plan and solution.

STANDARD 15. LEADERSHIP

The registered nurse provides leadership in the professional practice setting and the profession.

Measurement Criteria:

The registered nurse:

Engages in teamwork as a team player and a team builder.

Works to create and maintain healthy work environments in local, regional, national, or international communities.

Displays the ability to define a clear vision, the associated goals, and a plan to implement and measure progress.

Demonstrates a commitment to continuous, lifelong learning for self and others.

Teaches others to succeed by mentoring and other strategies.

Exhibits creativity and flexibility through times of change.

Demonstrates energy, excitement, and a passion for quality work.

Willingly accepts mistakes by self and others, thereby creating a culture in which risk-taking is not only safe, but expected.

Inspires loyalty through valuing of people as the most precious asset in an organization.

Directs the coordination of care across settings and among caregivers, including oversight of licensed and unlicensed personnel in any assigned or delegated tasks.

Serves in key roles in the work setting by participating on committees, councils, and administrative teams.

Promotes advancement of the profession through participation in professional organizations.

Additional Measurement Criteria for the Advanced Practice Registered Nurse:

The advanced practice registered nurse:

Works to influence decision-making bodies to improve patient care.

Provides direction to enhance the effectiveness of the healthcare team.

Initiates and revises protocols or guidelines to reflect evidence-based practice, to reflect accepted changes in care management, or to address emerging problems.

Promotes communication of information and advancement of the profession through writing, publishing, and presentations for professional or lay audiences.

Designs innovations to effect change in practice and improve health outcomes.

Additional Measurement Criteria for the Nursing Role Specialty:

The registered nurse in a nursing role specialty:

Works to influence decision-making bodies to improve patient care, health services, and policies.

Promotes communication of information and advancement of the profession through writing, publishing, and presentations for professional or lay audiences.

Designs innovations to effect change in practice and outcomes.

Provides direction to enhance the effectiveness of the multidisciplinary or interdisciplinary team.

GLOSSARY

Assessment. A systematic, dynamic process by which the registered nurse, through interaction with the patient, family, groups, communities, populations, and healthcare providers, collects and analyzes data. Assessment may include the following dimensions: physical, psychological, socio-cultural, spiritual, cognitive, functional abilities, developmental, economic, and lifestyle.

Caregiver. A person who provides direct care for another, such as a child, dependent adult, the disabled, or the chronically ill.

Code of ethics. A list of provisions that makes explicit the primary goals, values, and obligations of the profession.

Continuity of care. An interdisciplinary process that includes patients, families, and significant others in the development of a coordinated plan of care. This process facilitates the patient's transition between settings and healthcare providers, based on changing needs and available resources.

Criteria. Relevant, measurable indicators of the standards of practice and professional performance.

Data. Discrete entities that are described objectively without interpretation.

Diagnosis. A clinical judgment about the patient's response to actual or potential health conditions or needs. The diagnosis provides the basis for determination of a plan to achieve expected outcomes. Registered nurses utilize nursing and/or medical diagnoses depending upon educational and clinical preparation and legal authority.

Disease. A biological or psychosocial disorder of structure or function in a patient, especially one that produces specific signs or symptoms or that affects a specific part of the body, mind, or spirit.

Environment. The atmosphere, milieu, or conditions in which an individual lives, works, or plays.

Evaluation. The process of determining the progress toward attainment of expected outcomes. Outcomes include the effectiveness of care, when addressing one's practice.

Expected outcomes. End results that are measurable, desirable, and observable, and translate into observable behaviors.

Evidence-based practice. A process founded on the collection, interpretation, and integration of valid, important, and applicable patient-reported, clinician-observed, and research-derived evidence. The best available evidence, moderated by patient circumstances and preferences, is applied to improve the quality of clinical judgments.

Family. Family of origin or significant others as identified by the patient.

Guidelines. Systematically developed statements that describe recommended actions based on available scientific evidence and expert opinion. Clinical guidelines describe a process of patient care management that has the potential of improving the quality of clinical and consumer decision-making.

Health. An experience that is often expressed in terms of wellness and illness, and may occur in the presence or absence of disease or injury.

Healthcare providers. Individuals with special expertise who provide healthcare services or assistance to patients. They may include nurses, physicians, psychologists, social workers, nutritionists/dietitians, and various therapists.

Holistic. Based on an understanding that patient is an interconnected unity and that physical, mental, social, and spiritual factors need to be included in any interventions. The whole is a system that is greater than the sum of its parts.

Illness. The subjective experience of discomfort.

Implementation. Activities such as teaching, monitoring, providing, counseling, delegating, and coordinating.

Information. Data that are interpreted, organized, or structured.

Interdisciplinary. Reliant on the overlapping skills and knowledge of each team member and discipline, resulting in synergistic effects where outcomes are enhanced and more comprehensive than the simple aggregation of any team member's individual efforts.

Knowledge. Information that is synthesized so that relationships are identified and formalized.

Multidisciplinary. Reliant on each team member or discipline contributing discipline-specific skills.

Patient. Recipient of nursing practice. The term *patient* is used to provide consistency and brevity, bearing in mind that other terms, such as *client, individual, resident, family, groups, communities,* or *populations,* might be better choices in some instances. When the patient is an individual, the focus is on the health state, problems, or needs of the individual. When the patient is a family or group, the focus is on the health state of the unit as a whole or the reciprocal effects of the individual's health state on the other members of the unit. When the patient is a community or population, the focus is on personal and environmental health and the health risks of the community or population.

Peer review. A collegial, systematic, and periodic process by which registered nurses are held accountable for practice and which fosters the refinement of one's knowledge, skills, and decision-making at all levels and in all areas of practice.

Plan. A comprehensive outline of the components that need to be addressed to attain expected outcomes.

Quality of care. The degree to which health services for patients, families, groups, communities, or populations increase the likelihood of desired outcomes, and are consistent with current professional knowledge.

Situation. A set of circumstances, conditions, or events.

Standard. An authoritative statement defined and promoted by the profession by which the quality of practice, service, or education can be evaluated.

Strategy. A plan of action to achieve a major overall goal.

REFERENCES

Aiken, L. H., Clarke, S. P., Sloane, D. M., Sochalski, J., & Silber, J. H. (2002). Hospital registered nurse staffing and patient mortality, nurse burnout, and job dissatisfaction. *The Journal of the American Medical Association, 288* (16), 1987–1993.

American Nurses Association. (2003). *Nursing's social policy statement.* Washington, DC: Nursesbooks.org.

American Nurses Association. (2002). *Nursing's agenda for the future: A call to the nation.* Washington, DC: American Nurses Association.

American Nurses Association. (2001). *Code of ethics for nursing with interpretive statements.* Washington, DC: American Nurses Publishing.

American Nurses Association. (1998). *Standards of clinical nursing practice, 2nd edition.* Washington, DC: American Nurses Publishing.

American Nurses Association. (1996). *Scope and standards of advanced practice registered nursing.* Washington, DC: American Nurses Publishing.

American Nurses Association. (1995). *Nursing's social policy statement.* Washington, DC: American Nurses Publishing.

American Nurses Association. (1991). *Standards of clinical nursing practice.* Washington, DC: American Nurses Publishing.

American Nurses Association. (1987). *The scope of nursing practice.* Kansas City, MO: American Nurses Publishing.

American Nurses Association. (1973). *Standards of nursing practice.* Kansas City, MO: American Nurses Association.

Benner, P. (1982). From novice to expert. *American Journal of Nursing*, 82(3), 402–407

Chaffee, M. W., & Mills, M. E. C. (2001). Navy medicine: A health care leadership blueprint for the future. *Military Medicine,* 166 (3), 240–247.

George, J. (2002) *Nursing theories: The base for professional nursing practice.* Upper Saddle River, NJ: Prentice Hall.

Grant, A. B., and Massey, V. H. (1999). *Nursing leadership, management and research.* Springhouse, PA: Springhouse Corporation.

Institute of Medicine. (2000). *To err is human: Building a safer health system.* Washington, DC: National Academy Press.

Institute of Medicine. (2001). *Crossing the quality chasm: A new health system for the 21st century.* Summary. Washington, DC: National Academy Press. 2–4.

Kennedy, R. (2003). The nursing shortage and the role of technology. *Nursing Outlook*, 51, 533–534.

Needleman, J., and Buerhaus, P. (2003). Nurse staffing and patient safety: Current knowledge and implications for action. *International Journal for Quality in Health Care*, 15(4), 275–277.

Nightingale, F. (1859; reprinted 1926). *Notes on nursing: What it is, and what it is not.* New York: D. Appleton and Company

U.S. Department of Health and Human Services. (2002). *The registered nurse population: Findings from the National Sample Survey of Registered Nurses, March 2000.* Washington, DC: Health Resources and Services Administration, Bureau of Health Professions, Division of Nursing.

Appendix A
Timeline of the Development of Foundational Nursing Documents

The American Nurses Association has long been instrumental in the development of three foundational documents for professional nursing—a code of ethics, a scope and standards of practice, and a social policy statement. Each document contributes to understanding the context of nursing practice at the time of publication, and reflects the history of the evolution of the nursing profession in the United States.

Advancing communication technologies have expanded the revision process to permit ever increasing numbers of registered nurses to contribute to the open dialogue and review activities. This ensures the final published versions not only codify the consensus of the profession at the time of publication, but also reflect the experiences of those working in the profession at all levels and in all settings.

1859	Florence Nightingale publishes *Notes on Nursing: What It Is and What It Is Not.*
1896	The Nurses' Associated Alumnae of the United States and Canada is founded. Later to become the American Nurses Association (ANA), its first purpose is to establish and maintain a code of ethics.
1940	A "Tentative Code" is published in *American Journal of Nursing,* although never formally adopted.
1950	*Code for Professional Nurses,* in the form of 17 provisions that are a substantive revision of the "Tentative Code" of 1940, is unanimously accepted by the ANA House of Delegates.
1952	*Nursing Research* publishes its premiere issue.
1956	*Code for Professional Nurses* is amended.
1960	*Code for Professional Nurses* is revised.
1968	*Code for Professional Nurses* is substantively revised, condensing the 17 provisions of the 1960 Code into 10 provisions.
1973	ANA publishes its first *Standards of Nursing Practice.* (See Appendix B for a reproduction of this text.)
1976	*Code for Nurses with Interpretive Statements,* a modification of the provisions and interpretive statements, is published as 11 provisions.
1980	ANA publishes *Nursing: A Social Policy Statement.*
1985	The National Institutes of Health organizes the National Center for Nursing Research. ANA publishes *Titling for Licensure.* *Code for Nurses with Interpretive Statements* retains the provisions of the 1976 version and includes revised interpretive statements. The ANA House of Delegates forms a task force to formally document the scope of practice for nursing.

Foundational Nursing Documents

1987	ANA publishes *The Scope of Nursing Practice*. (See Appendix B for a reproduction of this text.)
1990	The ANA House of Delegates forms a task force to revise the 1973 *Standards of Nursing Practice*. (See Appendix C for a reproduction of this text.)
1991	ANA publishes *Standards of Clinical Nursing Practice*. (See Appendix D for a reproduction of this text.)
1995	ANA publishes *Nursing's Social Policy Statement*.
1995	The Congress of Nursing Practice directs the Committee on Nursing Practice Standards and Guidelines to establish a process for periodic review and revision of nursing standards.
1996	ANA publishes *Scope and Standards of Advanced Practice Registered Nursing*.
1998	ANA publishes *Standards of Clinical Nursing Practice, 2nd Edition*, (also known as the *Clinical Standards*. (See Appendix E for a reproduction of this text.)
2001	*Code of Ethics for Nurses with Interpretive Statements* is accepted by the ANA House of Delegates. ANA publishes *Bill of Rights for Registered Nurses*.
2002	ANA publishes *Nursing's Agenda for the Future: A Call to the Nation*.
2003	ANA publishes *Nursing's Social Policy Statement, 2nd Edition*. ANA publishes *Nursing: Scope and Standards of Practice*.

APPENDIX B
Standards of Nursing Practice (1973)

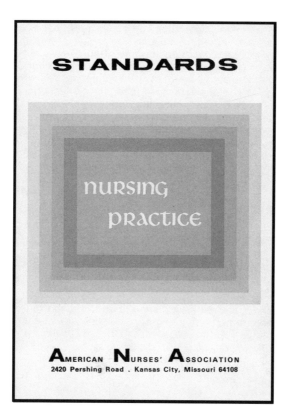

STANDARDS OF NURSING PRACTICE

Nursing practice is a direct service, goal directed and adaptable to the needs of the individual, family and community during health and illness. Professional practitioners of nursing bear primary responsibility and accountability for the nursing care clients/patients receive. The purpose of Standards of Nursing Practice is to fulfill the profession's obligation to provide and improve this practice.

The Standards focus on practice. They provide a means for determining the quality of nursing which a client/patient receives regardless of whether such services are provided solely by a professional nurse or by a professional nurse and nonprofessional assistants.

The Standards are stated according to a systematic approach to nursing practice: the assessment of the client's/patient's status, the plan of nursing actions, the implementation of the plan, and the evaluation. These specific divisions are not intended to imply that practice consists of a series of discrete steps, taken in strict sequence, beginning with assessment and ending with evaluation. The processes described are used concurrently and recurrently. Assessment, for example, frequently continues during implementation; similarly, evaluation dictates reassessment and replanning.

These Standards for Nursing Practice apply to nursing practice in any setting. Nursing practice in all settings must possess the characteristics identified by these Standards if clients/patients are to receive a high quality of nursing care. Each Standard is followed by a rationale and assessment factors. Assessment factors are to be used in determining achievement of the Standard.

STANDARD I

THE COLLECTION OF DATA ABOUT THE HEALTH STATUS OF THE CLIENT/PATIENT IS SYSTEMATIC AND CONTINUOUS. THE DATA ARE ACCESSIBLE, COMMUNICATED, AND RECORDED.

Rationale: Comprehensive care requires complete and ongoing collection of data about the client/patient to determine the nursing care needs of the client/patient. All health status data about the client/patient must be available for all members of the health care team.

Assessment Factors:
1. Health status data include:
    —Growth and development
    —Biophysical status
    —Emotional status
    —Cultural, religious, socioeconomic background
    —Performance of activities of daily living
    —Patterns of coping
    —Interaction patterns
    —Client's/patient's perception of and satisfaction with his health status
    —Client/patient health goals
    —Environment (physical, social, emotional, ecological)
    —Available and accessible human and material resources
2. Data are collected from:
    —Client/patient, family, significant others
    —Health care personnel
    —Individuals within the immediate environment and/or the community

3. Data are obtained by:
   —Interview
   —Examination
   —Observation
   —Reading records, reports, etc.
4. There is a format for the collection of data which:
   —Provides for a systematic collection of data
   —Facilitates the completeness of data collection
5. Continuous collection of data is evident by:
   —Frequent updating
   —Recording of changes in health status
6. The data are:
   —Accessible on the client/patient records
   —Retrievable from record-keeping systems
   —Confidential when appropriate

STANDARD II
NURSING DIAGNOSES ARE DERIVED FROM HEALTH STATUS DATA.

Rationale: The health status of the client/patient is the basis for determining the nursing care needs. The data are analyzed and compared to norms when possible.

Assessment Factors:
1. The client's/patient's health status is compared to the norm in order to determine if there is a deviation from the norm and the degree and direction of deviation.
2. The client's/patient's capabilities and limitations are identified.
3. The nursing diagnoses are related to and congruent with the diagnoses of all other professionals caring for the client/patient.

STANDARD III
THE PLAN OF NURSING CARE INCLUDES GOALS DERIVED FROM THE NURSING DIAGNOSES.

Rationale: The determination of the results to be achieved is an essential part of planning care.

Assessment Factors:
1. Goals are mutually set with the client/patient and pertinent others:
   —They are congruent with other planned therapies.
   —They are stated in realistic and measurable terms.
   —They are assigned a time period for achievement.
2. Goals are established to maximize functional capabilities and are congruent with:
   —Growth and development
   —Biophysical status
   —Behavioral patterns
   —Human and material resources

STANDARD IV
THE PLAN OF NURSING CARE INCLUDES PRIORITIES AND THE PRESCRIBED NURSING APPROACHES OR MEASURES TO ACHIEVE THE GOALS DERIVED FROM THE NURSING DIAGNOSES.

Rationale: Nursing actions are planned to promote, maintain and restore the client's/patient's well-being.

Assessment Factors:
1. Physiological measures are planned to manage (prevent or control) specific patient problems and are related to the nursing diagnoses and goals of care, e.g. ADL, use of self-help devices, etc.
2. Psychosocial measures are specific to the client's/patient's nursing care problem and to the nursing care goals, e.g. techniques to control aggression, motivation.
3. Teaching-learning principles are incorporated into the plan of care and objectives for learning stated in behavioral terms, e.g. specification of content for learner's level, reinforcement, readiness, etc.

Appendix B: Standards of Nursing Practice (1973)   **59**

4. Approaches are planned to provide for a therapeutic environment:
    —Physical environmental factors are used to influence the therapeutic environment, e.g. control of noise, control of temperature, etc.
    —Psychosocial measures are used to structure the environment for therapeutic ends, e.g. paternal participation in all phases of the maternity experience.
    —Group behaviors are used to structure interaction and influence the therapeutic environment, e.g. conformity, ethos, territorial rights, locomotion, etc.
5. Approaches are specified for orientation of the client/patient to:
    —New roles and relationships
    —Relevant health (human and material) resources.
    —Modifications in plan of nursing care
    —Relationship of modifications in nursing care plan to the total care plan
6. The plan of nursing care includes the utilization of available and appropriate resources:
    —Human resources — other health personnel
    —Material resources
    —Community
7. The plan includes an ordered sequence of nursing actions.
8. Nursing approaches are planned on the basis of current scientific knowledge.

STANDARD V

NURSING ACTIONS PROVIDE FOR CLIENT/PATIENT PARTICIPATION IN HEALTH PROMOTION, MAINTENANCE AND RESTORATION.

Rationale: The client/patient and family are continually involved in nursing care.

Assessment Factors:
1. The client/patient and family are kept informed about:
    —Current health status
    —Changes in health status
    —Total health care plan
    —Nursing care plan
    —Roles of health care personnel
    —Health care resources
2. The client/patient and family are provided with the information needed to make decisions and choices about:
    —Promoting, maintaining and restoring health
    —Seeking and utilizing appropriate health care personnel
    —Maintaining and using health care resources

STANDARD VI

NURSING ACTIONS ASSIST THE CLIENT/PATIENT TO MAXIMIZE HIS HEALTH CAPABILITIES.

Rationale: Nursing actions are designed to promote, maintain and restore health.

Assessment Factors:
1. Nursing actions:
    —Are consistent with the plan of care.
    —Are based on scientific principles.
    —Are individualized to the specific situation.
    —Are used to provide a safe and therapeutic environment.
    —Employ teaching-learning opportunities for the client/patient.
    —Include utilization of appropriate resources.
2. Nursing actions are directed by the client's/patient's physical, physiological, psychological and social behavior associated with:
    —Ingestion of food, fluid and nutrients
    —Elimination of body wastes and excesses in fluid

—Locomotion and exercise
—Regulatory mechanisms—body heat, metabolism.
—Relating to others
—Self-actualization

STANDARD VII

THE CLIENT'S/PATIENT'S PROGRESS OR LACK OF PROGRESS TOWARD GOAL ACHIEVEMENT IS DETERMINED BY THE CLIENT/PATIENT AND THE NURSE.

Rationale: The quality of nursing care depends upon comprehensive and intelligent determination of nursing's impact upon the health status of the client/patient. The client/patient is an essential part of this determination.

Assessment Factors:

1. Current data about the client/patient are used to measure his progress toward goal achievement.
2. Nursing actions are analyzed for their effectiveness in the goal achievement of the client/patient.
3. The client/patient evaluates nursing actions and goal achievement.
4. Provision is made for nursing follow-up of a particular client/patient to determine the long-term effects of nursing care.

STANDARD VIII

THE CLIENT'S/PATIENT'S PROGRESS OR LACK OF PROGRESS TOWARD GOAL ACHIEVEMENT DIRECTS REASSESSMENT, REORDERING OF PRIORITIES, NEW GOAL SETTING AND REVISION OF THE PLAN OF NURSING CARE.

Rationale: The nursing process remains the same, but the input of new information may dictate new or revised approaches.

Assessment Factors:

1. Reassessment is directed by goal achievement or lack of goal achievement.
2. New priorities and goals are determined and additional nursing approaches are prescribed appropriately.
3. New nursing actions are accurately and appropriately initiated.

WHY STANDARDS OF PRACTICE?

"A professional association is an organization of practitioners who judge one another a
professionally competent and who have banded together to perform social functions whic
they cannot perform in their separate capacity as individuals."[1]

A professional association, because of its nature, must provide measures to judge th
competency of its membership and to evaluate the quality of its services. Studies show tha
the tendency for self-organization has been found to be characteristic of professions and th
establishment and implementation of standards characteristic of the organization. Mary Folle
points out that professional associations have one function above all others:

"The members do not come together merely for the pleasure of meeting others of the sam
occupation; nor do they meet primarily to increase their pecuniary gain; although this ma
be one of the objects. They join in order to better perform their functions. They meet:

To establish standards.
To maintain standards.
To improve standards.
To keep members up to standards.
To educate the public to appreciate standards.
To protect the public from those individuals who have not attained standards o
willfully do not follow them.
To protect individual members of the profession from each other."[2]

A profession's concern for the quality of its service constitutes the heart of its responsibili
to the public. The more expertise required to perform the service, the greater is society
dependence upon those who carry it out. A profession must seek control of its practice i
order to guarantee the quality of its service to the public. Behind that guarantee are th
standards of the profession that provide the assurance that the guarantee will be met. Th
is essential both for the protection of the public and the profession itself. A profession tha
does not maintain the confidence of the public will soon cease to be a social force.

In recognition of the importance of standards of professional practice and the need t
guarantee quality service, the various Divisions on Practice have each formulated a set o
standards. The American Nurses' Association recognizes that as standards are implemente
in practice settings and as the scope of nursing practice enlarges and the theoretical bas
upon which this practice rests becomes more sharply delineated, ongoing revision of th
standards of professional practice will be warranted.

Congress for Nursing Practice

---

[1] Merton, Robert K. "The Functions of the Professional Association" **American Journal of Nursing**, Vol. 5
(January, 1958), p. 50.

[2] **Dynamic Administration**, The Collected Papers of Mary Follet edited by Henry C. Metcalf and L. Urwic
New York: Harper & Brothers, 1942, p. 136.

APPENDIX C
The Scope of Nursing Practice (1987)

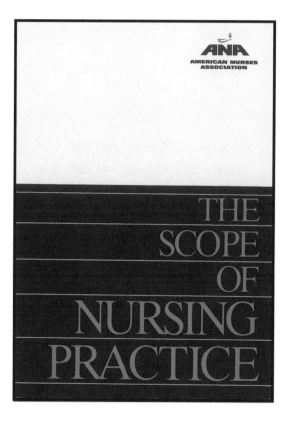

Contents

Introduction

The 1985 House of Delegates of the American Nurses Association directed ANA's Cabinets on Nursing Education, Practice, and Services to jointly delineate the future scope of practice for persons educated with a baccalaureate or higher degree in nursing and for those educated with an associate degree in nursing. The Task Force on Scope of Practice was formed to address the charge of the House of Delegates. The task force report was received by the ANA Board of Directors and forwarded as amended to the 1987 ANA House of Delegates. The House of Delegates then amended and adopted the report as the position of the American Nurses Association.

In its deliberations, the task force clarified the differences between two concepts: the scope of practice and the nature of nursing. The task force concluded that the nature of nursing and its unique contribution to society had been described in *Nursing: A Social Policy Statement.*[1]

The social policy statement describes the nature of nursing as complex and highly interactive, and asserts that society has historically understood nursing to be a non-invasive, nurturing discipline, focused more on creating the physiological, psychological, and sociocultural environment in which the patient can gain or maintain health or heal than on the diagnosis and treatment of disease.

The task force also noted that various ANA documents had described the nature of nursing as a scholarly discipline,[2] the nature of nursing education,[3] the nature of nursing administration,[4, 5] and the nature of specialization.[6, 7]

The task force decided that this document, the ANA *Statement on the Scope of Nursing Practice,* ought to focus exclusively on the dynamic scope of the clinical practice of nursing. The characteristics of that scope of clinical practice are defined in this report.

The Single Scope
of Clinical Nursing Practice

There is one scope of clinical nursing practice. The core, or essence, of that practice is the nursing diagnosis and treatment of human responses to health and to illness. This core of the clinical practice of nursing is dynamic, and evolves as patterns of human response amenable to nursing intervention are identified, nursing diagnoses are forumulated and classified, nursing skills and patterns of intervention are made more explicit, and patient outcomes responsive to nursing intervention are evaluated.

Differences between the Professional
and Technical Practice of Nursing

The depth and breadth to which the individual nurse engages in the total scope of the clinical practice of nursing are defined by the knowledge base of the nurse, the role of the nurse, and the nature of the client population within a practice environment. In the future, these same characteristics will differentiate the professional and technical practice of nursing.

Knowledge Base of the Nurse

Differences between the knowledge base for professional and technical nursing practice are both quantitative and qualitative. Education for professional practice is provided within baccalaureate or higher degree programs with a major in nursing. Set within the framework of liberal education, these programs provide for the study of nursing theory within the context of related scientific, behavioral, and humanistic disciplines. Graduates of professional programs have the knowledge base requisite for additional formal education in specialized clinical practice, nursing research, nursing administration, and nursing education.

Graduates of professional programs are prepared to engage in the full scope of the clinical practice of nursing. They must be educated to understand the various modes of nursing inquiry and the principles of scientific investigation, and must be able to synthesize relevant information and make clinical inferences. They must know how to project patient outcomes, establish nursing plans of care to achieve those outcomes, and evaluate the patient's response to nursing intervention. They must apply nursing theory to the assessment, diagnosis, treatment, and evaluation of human responses to health and illness in both the individual clinical situation and the broader community setting.

Education for the technical practice of nursing is provided in community colleges or other institutions of higher education qualified to offer the associate degree in nursing. Set within the framework of general education, these programs provide for the study of nursing within the context of the applied sciences. Clinical content is empirical in nature and focuses on skills, facts, demonstrated relationships, and experimentally verified observations.

Graduates of associate degree programs are prepared to engage in the technical aspects of the clinical practice of nursing. They must have the knowledge base to apply a circumscribed body of established nursing principles and skills. They must be educated to understand patient problems from a biological, social, and psychological perspective, and to use a problem-solving approach to the health care of individuals and their families in a variety of organzied nursing service settings.

Role of the Nurse

Professional nurses in clinical practice function as direct care givers in both institutional and community settings. In addition, professional nurses function as clinical specialists, as patient care managers, as clinical educators, as clinical researchers, and as case managers or coordinators of patient care services within the broader health service system. Professional nurses collaborate with health care colleagues and provide direction to the technical nurse.

Professional nurses develop nursing policies, procedures, and protocols, and set standards of practice for nursing care for all client populations in all practice settings. Professional nurses assess human responses to health and illness, formulate nursing diagnoses, explicate nursing interventions, and direct and evaluate nursing practice.

Technical nurses function primarily as direct care givers within organized nursing services and use a problem-solving approach to the care of individuals and their families in institutional and community settings. Technical nurses use policies, procedures, and protocols developed by professional nurses in implementing an individual's plan of care. Technical nurses are accountable for practicing within these guidelines.

Nature of the Client Population
Within the Practice Environment

The scope of clinical practice in which the professional nurse may engage is limited only by the depth and breadth to which the profession has evolved, and is not further limited by the nature of the client population or the practice environment.

The scope of clinical practice in which the technical nurse may engage is limited to the application of the circumscribed body of nursing principles and skills established by the profession for defined patient populations.

Technical nurses practice in settings in which nursing is controlled through mechanisms such as organized nursing services, professional nursing staff structures, and professional nursing standards, policies, procedures, and protocols.

Professional and Legal Regulation of Practice

Nursing, like other professions, is accountable for ensuring that its members act in the public interest by providing the unique service society has entrusted to them. The process by which the profession does this is called professional regulation, or self-regulation. Nursing regulates itself by defining its practice base, providing for research and development of that practice base, establishing a system for nursing education, establishing the structures through which nursing services will be delivered, and providing quality assurance mechanisms such as a code of ethics, standards of practice, structures for peer review, and a system of credentialing. Professional nursing is accountable to derive standards of practice for defined patient populations in specific practice environments.

The legal contract between society and the recognized professions is spelled out in statute. Legal regulation is the process by which the state attests to the public that the individual licensed to practice is at least minimally competent to practice.

Figure 1 illustrates the parallel relationships of the component parts of professional and legal regulation of nursing practice.

The professional regulation of nursing practice, as Figure 1 indicates, is based on the profession's definition of the nature and scope of nursing practice. Professional standards evolve from the scope of nursing practice. Standards provide the framework for the development of competency statements as well as for statements of educational outcomes and standards for organized

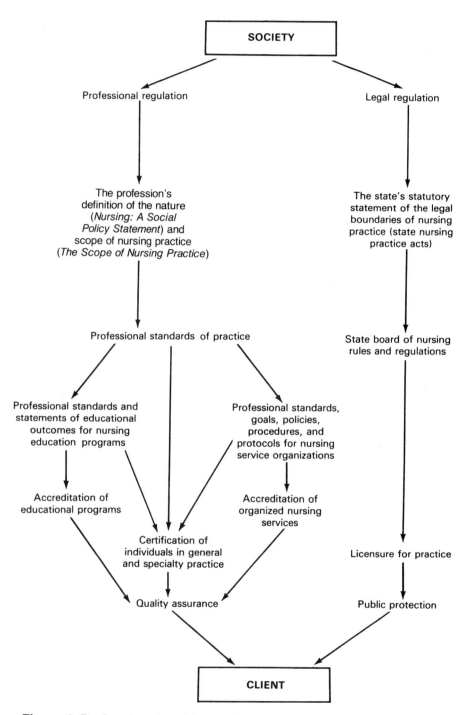

Figure 1. Professional and Legal Regulation of Nursing Practice.

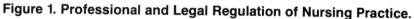

nursing services. The profession also uses its standards in the accreditation and certification processes that lead to quality assurance for the client.

The legal regulation of nursing practice is based on the definition of nursing in nursing practice acts. Legal boundaries are derived from this definition of nursing and are used to provide the basis for interpretation of the safe practice of nursing. Rules and regulations evolve from these acts and are the guidelines used by state boards of nursing to issue licenses and ensure the public safety. The statutory definition of nursing needs to encompass the profession's definition of its practice base, and to be not only general enough to provide for nursing's dynamic nature and evolving practice, but also specific enough to differentiate the professional and technical practice of nursing and to differentiate nursing from other statutorily regulated health professions.

Historical Overview

Following a request from its 1964 House of Delegates, ANA identified two categories of nursing practice and delineated the educational preparation for each category. The minimum preparation for beginning professional nursing practice was identified as baccalaureate education in nursing, and the minimum preparation for beginning technical nursing practice was identified as associate degree education in nursing. *Educational Preparation for Nurse Practitioners and Assistants to Nurses: A Position Paper*, published by ANA in 1965, described the two categories and the educational preparation appropriate to each category.[8]

The 1978 House of Delegates charged the association with deriving a comprehensive statement of competencies for the two categories of nursing practice.[9] The Commission on Nursing Education formed the Ad Hoc Competency Work Group, which gave the 1980 House of Delegates a lengthy report listing selected competencies for baccalaureate-prepared and associate-degree-prepared nurses, and making recommendations.[10] The 1980 House of Delegates resolved that a progress report on the development of a comprehensive statement of competencies should be presented to the 1982 House of Delegates.[11] The Commission on Nursing Education received a report from the Ad Hoc Competency Work Group in November 1981. The commission decided that "further efforts to describe nursing roles from a competency base could best be done in the practice setting. . . . Attempting to define nursing practice from a competency base instead of an educational base has not served to clarify two kinds of nursing practice."[12]

In 1984 and 1985, ANA reaffirmed the educational bases and established titles for two categories of nurses in the future. The educational bases are baccalaureate and associate degree preparation in nursing. The titles are *registered nurse* and *associate nurse*. The categories are professional and technical nursing practice.

The 1985 House of Delegates directed the Cabinets on Nursing Education, Practice, and Services to collaborate in delineating the scope of practice for future professional and technical nurses. The Task Force on Scope of Practice was appointed, consisting of representatives from the three cabinets and a consultant from the National Commission on Nursing Implementation Project. An informational report on the task force's progress, "Scope of Practice for Technical and Professional Nursing," was presented to the 1986 House of Delegates by the Cabinet on Nursing Education.

Several meetings were held in 1985, 1986, and 1987 to determine areas of agreement among the various sectors of organized nursing concerning the nursing profession's scope of practice. For example, in 1985 and 1987, ANA representatives met with representatives of the National Federation of Licensed Practical Nurses to clarify both organizations' positions regarding titling and licensing for nursing practice.

In 1986, chairpersons of all ANA cabinets met with the National League for Nursing's council chairpersons to plan for the implementation of two levels of nursing practice. In 1987, representatives of ANA, NLN, the American Association of Colleges of Nursing, the American Organization of Nurse Executives, and the National Commission on Nursing Implementation Project, and the chair of the ANA Task Force on Scope of Practice met to consider common organizational understandings concerning the scope of practice. Representatives of ANA, NLN, and the National Council of

State Boards of Nursing met to consider the implications of the profession's definition of its clinical scope of practice for licensure examinations.

Information upon which to base the statement on the scope of practice was collected, analyzed, and shared. All ANA cabinets, state nurses associations, participants in the Nursing Organization Liaison Forum, and other key nursing organizations participated in the field review of the scope of nursing practice statement. The National Commission on Nursing Implementation Project collected information developed by state nurses associations, ANA, NLN, AONE, NFLPN, and other organizations and groups regarding categories of nursing practice, and conducted an initial content analysis of the statements of competencies of nurses prepared with a baccalaureate in nursing and those with an associate degree in nursing. The American Association of Colleges of Nursing conducted a two-year project to define the essential elements of college and university education for professional nursing. The documents developed by these projects were shared with the relevant ANA cabinets and were instrumental in the task force's development of this scope of practice statement.

References

1. American Nurses Association. *Nursing: A Social Policy Statement*. Kansas City, Mo.: the Association, 1980.

2. American Nurses Association. Statement on Nursing Care Research. Kansas City, Mo., 1985, unpublished.

3. American Nurses Association. *Educational Preparation for Nurse Practitioners and Assistants to Nurses: A Position Paper*. Kansas City, Mo.: the Association, 1965.

4. American Nurses Association. *Standards for Organized Nursing Services*. Kansas City, Mo.: the Association, 1982.

5. American Nurses Association. *New Organizational Models and Financial Arrangements for Nursing Services*. Kansas City, Mo.: the Association, 1986.

6. American Nurses Association. *Nursing: A Social Policy Statement, op. cit.*

7. American Nurses Association. Specialization in Nursing Practice: Informational Report of Cabinet on Nursing Practice to 1985 House of Delegates. Kansas City, Mo., 1985, unpublished.

8. American Nurses Association. *Educational Preparation for Nurse Practitioners and Assistants to Nurses: A Position Paper*. New York: the Association, 1965, 6–8.

9. American Nurses Association. *Summary of Proceedings: 1978 Convention*. Kansas City, Mo.: the Association, 1979, 71.

10. American Nurses Association. *Summary of Proceedings: 1980 Convention*. Kansas City, Mo.: the Association, 1981, 275–288.

11. *Ibid.*, 85.

12. American Nurses Association. *Summary of Proceedings: 1982 Convention*. Kansas City, Mo.: the Association, 1983, 96.

APPENDIX D
Standards of Clinical Nursing Practice (1991)

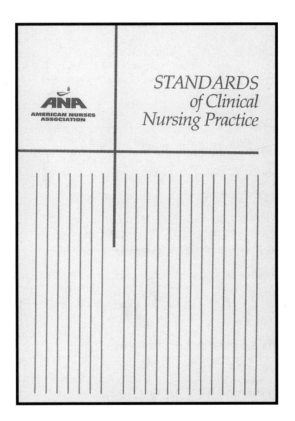

CONTENTS

PREFACE

The American Nurses Association (ANA) has actively engaged in standards development since the late 1960s. The first standards of practice for the nursing profession were published by ANA in 1973.[1] These standards were generic in nature and focused on the nursing process. Numerous specialty groups and organizations also have promulgated standards of nursing practice — some in collaboration with ANA and others independently. These standards have varied widely in their purposes, scopes, and formats. The divergent approaches previously used to develop nursing standards have limited their usefulness for nurses, other health care providers, payers, policymakers, and consumers of nursing services.

There are currently a number of activities occurring in health care that add new importance to the manner in which the profession addresses standards of nursing practice. Increases in health care costs, competition, and regulation are forcing health care providers to define their practice in a measurable way and to identify the client outcomes to which they contribute. Additionally, federal and private sector initiatives are focusing on the development of methods to evaluate the quality, appropriateness, and effectiveness of health care services. The nursing profession continues to closely monitor the evolving external environment and analyze the need to modify existing standards or develop new standards for all areas of nursing practice. Standards also must receive ongoing attention by the profession to assure that they remain timely and reflect advances in nursing knowledge and clinical technology.

In a report to the 1988 ANA House of Delegates, the ANA Cabinet on Nursing Practice and Council on Medical-Surgical Nursing Practice recommended that ANA formally clarify the nature, purpose, and promulgation of ANA standards of nursing practice. In 1989, a task force was appointed with the following charge:

> In view of current health care quality assurance activities, define the nature and purpose of standards of practice for nursing and the relationship of quality assurance activities and standards of practice to specialization in nursing practice, credentialing, and implications for nursing information systems.

As a part of the task force's 1990 report, it was recommended that the 1973 *Standards of Nursing Practice* be revised. The task force eventually became the Standing Committee on Nursing Practice Standards and Guidelines, under the ANA Congress of Nursing Practice. A subsequent Task Force on Nursing Practice Standards was then appointed to revise the 1973 standards.

In fulfilling its charge, the committee and task force were committed to working with specialty nursing organizations and groups. Numerous specialty organizations and groups have provided guidance and comment throughout this work. This collaborative effort has resulted in the development of standards that are applicable to all nurses engaged in clinical practice. Use of a common language and consistent format will both clarify and strengthen nursing's ability to articulate the scope of nursing practice across all clinical areas.

This publication sets forth standards of clinical nursing practice for the nursing profession and reflects the definitions, purpose and framework for standards and guidelines developed by the 1989 task force. This publication is intended to be used in conjunction with other documents that articulate the values of the nursing profession and the definition and scope of nursing practice.[2,3,4,5,6,7,8,9]

Standards are broad statements that address the full scope of professional nursing practice. The development of *Standards of Clinical Nursing Practice* occurred simultaneously with the development of practice guidelines. Guidelines are specific to a clinical condition (e.g., pain, urinary incontinence, pressure ulcers), and assist the nurse and others in clinical decision making by describing recommended courses of action for various clinical situations or specific client conditions or populations. Guidelines provide linkages among diagnoses or clinical conditions, interventions, and outcomes. They also describe alternatives available to each client or client population and provide a basis for the evaluation of care and allocation of resources.

Work on developing guidelines is underway by organized nursing. Nurses possessing a wealth of clinical expertise also are actively working with interdisciplinary groups to develop guidelines at the national level.

INTRODUCTION

Role of Standards

Standards are authoritative statements by which the nursing profession describes the responsibilities for which its practitioners are accountable. Consequently, standards reflect the values and priorities of the profession. Standards provide direction for professional nursing practice and a framework for the evaluation of practice. Written in measurable terms, standards also define the nursing profession's accountability to the public and the client outcomes for which nurses are responsible.

Development of Standards

Standards of professional nursing practice may pertain to general or specialty practice. A professional nursing organization has a responsibility to its membership and the public it serves to develop standards of practice. As the professional organization for all registered nurses, ANA is responsible for developing generic standards that apply to the practice of all professional nurses.

This publication sets forth standards of clinical nursing practice. It has been developed by ANA, in collaboration with numerous specialty nursing organizations and groups, for the nursing profession. *Standards of Clinical Nursing Practice* describes a competent level of professional nursing care and professional performance common to all nurses engaged in clinical practice.

Organizing Principles of *Standards of Clinical Nursing Practice*

Standards of Clinical Nursing Practice applies to the care that is provided to all clients. "Clients" may include an individual, family, group, or community for whom the nurse is providing formally specified services as sanctioned by nursing practice acts. This care may be provided in the context of disease or injury prevention, health promotion, health restoration, or health maintenance. The cultural, racial, and ethnic diversity of the client must always be taken into account in providing nursing services.

Standards of Clinical Nursing Practice is generic in nature and applies to all registered nurses engaged in clinical practice, regardless of clinical specialty, practice setting, or educational preparation.

Standards that further define the responsibilities of nurses engaged in specialty practice or nurses who function at advanced levels of clinical practice are determined by those nursing specialties and appropriate groups within ANA.

Professional nursing organizations and groups within ANA representing nurses practicing in specialty areas or functioning at advanced levels of practice (i.e., clinical specialists, nurse practitioners, nurse midwives, and nurse anesthetists) will develop standards by building on *Standards of Clinical Nursing Practice* to develop specific criteria for defining expectations associated with the area of clinical practice or role.[*] However, nurses practicing in a specialty area and/or nurses practicing at an advanced level of practice will be accountable for meeting the standards of clinical nursing practice.

Standards of Clinical Nursing Practice consists of "Standards of Care" and "Standards of Professional Performance," which include the following:

Standards of Care
- Assessment
- Diagnosis
- Outcome Identification
- Planning
- Implementation
- Evaluation

Standards of Professional Performance
- Quality of Care
- Performance Appraisal
- Education
- Collegiality
- Ethics
- Collaboration
- Research
- Resource Utilization

Standards of Care

"Standards of Care" describe a competent level of nursing care as demonstrated by the nursing process, involving assessment, diagnosis, outcome identification, planning, implementation, and evaluation. The

---

[*]Standards for nurses whose primary role is in an area such as research, education, or administration are described in other ANA publications.[2,3,4,5,6,7,8,9]

nursing process encompasses all significant actions taken by nurses in providing care to all clients, and forms the foundation of clinical decision making. Additional nursing responsibilities for all clients (such as providing culturally and ethnically relevant care, maintaining a safe environment, educating clients about their illness, treatment, health promotion or self-care activities, and planning for continuity of care) are subsumed within these standards. Therefore, "Standards of Care" delineate care that is provided to all clients of nursing services.

Standards of Professional Performance

"Standards of Professional Performance" describe a competent level of behavior in the professional role — including activities related to quality of care, performance appraisal, education, collegiality, ethics, collaboration, research, and resource utilization. All nurses are expected to engage in professional role activities appropriate to their education, position, and practice setting. While this is an assumption of all of the "Standards of Professional Performance", the scope of nursing involvement in some professional roles is particularly dependent upon the nurse's education, position, and practice environment. Therefore, some standards or measurement criteria identify a broad range of activities that may demonstrate compliance with the standard.

Standards for specialty or advanced practice may elaborate on appropriate expectations for the various professional role standards. These standards would be generated by the appropriate specialty group or organization.

While "Standards of Professional Performance" describe roles expected of all professional nurses, many other responsibilities comprise the hallmarks of a profession. The nurse should be self-directed and purposeful in seeking necessary knowledge and skills to enhance career goals. Other activities — such as membership in a professional nursing organization, certification in specialty or advanced practice, and further academic education — are desirable methods to enhance the nurse's professionalism.

Criteria

Standards of Clinical Nursing Practice includes criteria that allow the standards to be measured. Criteria include key indicators of competent practice. For the most part, standards should remain stable over time, as they reflect the philosophical values of the profession. However, criteria should be revised to incorporate advancements in scientific knowledge, clinical practice, and technology. Criteria must remain consonant with current nursing practice, which has a theoretical basis but is constantly evolving through the development of new knowledge and incorporation of relevant research findings into aspects of the nursing process.

Assumptions

Standards of Clinical Nursing Practice focuses primarily on the process of providing nursing care and performing professional role activities. These standards apply to all nurses in all areas of clinical practice despite the tremendous variability in environments in which nurses practice. However, it is important to recognize the link between working conditions and the nurse's ability to deliver care. It is the responsibility of employers or health care facilities to provide an appropriate environment for nursing practice.

Although it is the nurse's responsibility to meet these standards, *Standards of Clinical Nursing Practice* assumes that adequate environmental working conditions and necessary resources are available to support and facilitate the nurse's attainment of nursing practice standards. Related standards that address the work environment are found in other ANA publications.[2,3,4,5,6,7,8,9] These other publications and *Standards of Clinical Nursing Practice* can be used to determine the resources necessary to provide an adequate work environment. In addition, nurses in specialty areas or nontraditional settings may benefit from having structural criteria clearly defined within the standards of specialty organizations.

Several related themes underlie *Standards of Clinical Nursing Practice*. Nursing care must be individualized to meet a particular client's unique needs and situation. The nurse also must respect the client's goals and preferences in developing and implementing a plan of care. Given that one of the nurse's primary responsibilities is client education, nurses must provide clients with appropriate information to make informed decisions regarding their health care and treatment, including health promotion and prevention of disease. However, it is recognized that some state regulations or institutional policies or procedures may prohibit full disclosure of information to clients or may require reporting of confidential information.

Standards of Clinical Nursing Practice also recognizes the nurse's partnership with the client and other health care providers. These standards assume that the nurse works with other health care providers in a coordinated manner throughout the process of rendering care to a client. In addition, the involvement of the client, the family, or significant others is seen as paramount. Of course, the appropriate degree of participation expected of the client, the family, or other health care providers must be inferred from the clinical environment and client's unique situation.

Throughout this document, terms such as "appropriate", "pertinent," and "realistic" are used. It is beyond the scope of a document such as this to account for all possible scenarios that the professional nurse may encounter in clinical practice. It is expected that with the development of criteria for areas of specialty practice, more specific details about expectations will be outlined. However, even with the addition of specialty area criteria, the nurse will need to exercise judgment based on education and experience in determining what is appropriate, pertinent, or realistic. Further direction may be available from documents such as guidelines for practice or agency standards, policies, procedures, and protocols.

Summary

Standards of Clinical Nursing Practice delineates the professional responsibilities of all registered nurses engaged in clinical practice regardless of setting. *Standards of Clinical Nursing Practice* and nursing practice guidelines could serve as a basis for:

- quality assurance systems;
- data bases;
- regulatory systems;
- health care reimbursement and financing methodologies;
- development and evaluation of nursing service delivery systems and organizational structures;
- certification activities;
- job descriptions and performance appraisals;
- agency policies, procedures, and protocols; and
- educational offerings.

In order to best serve the public health and the nursing profession, nursing must continue efforts to develop standards of practice and practice guidelines. Nursing must examine how standards and practice guidelines can be disseminated and used most effectively to enhance and promote the quality of clinical practice. In addition, standards and practice guidelines must be evaluated on an ongoing basis, with revisions made as necessary. The dynamic nature of the health care environment and the growing body of nursing research provide both the impetus and the means by which nursing will proactively respond to ensure competent clinical practice and promote ongoing professional development and client care.

KEY TERMS

Definitions of key terms will assist in using this document. Other definitions are found in the Glossary at the end of this publication.

ASSESSMENT. A systematic, dynamic process by which the nurse, through interaction with the client, significant others, and health care providers, collects and analyzes data about the client. Data may include the following dimensions: physical, psychological, sociocultural, spiritual, cognitive, functional abilities, developmental, economic, and life-style.

DIAGNOSIS. A clinical judgment about the client's response to actual or potential health conditions or needs. Diagnoses provide the basis for determination of a plan of care to achieve expected outcomes.

EVALUATION. The process of determining both the client's progress toward the attainment of expected outcomes and the effectiveness of nursing care.

IMPLEMENTATION. May include any or all of these activities: intervening, delegating, coordinating. The client, significant others, or health care providers may be designated to implement interventions within the plan of care.

OUTCOMES. Measurable, expected, client-focused goals.

PLAN OF CARE. Comprehensive outline of care to be delivered to attain expected outcomes.

CLIENT. Recipient of nursing actions. When the client is an individual, the focus is on the health state, problems, or needs of a single person. When the client is a family or group, the focus is on the health state of the unit as a whole or the reciprocal effects of an individual's health state on the other members of the unit. When the client is a community, the focus is on personal and environmental health and the health risks of population groups. Nursing actions toward clients may be directed to disease or injury prevention, health promotion, health restoration, or health maintenance.

HEALTH CARE PROVIDERS. Individuals with special expertise who provide health care services or assistance to clients. They may include nurses, physicians, psychologists, social workers, nutritionists/dieticians, and various therapists. Providers also may include service organizations and vendors.

SIGNIFICANT OTHERS. Family members and/or those significant to the client.

STANDARDS OF CARE

Standard I. Assessment

THE NURSE COLLECTS CLIENT HEALTH DATA.

Measurement Criteria

1. The priority of data collection is determined by the client's immediate condition or needs.
2. Pertinent data are collected using appropriate assessment techniques.
3. Data collection involves the client, significant others, and health care providers when appropriate.
4. The data collection process is systematic and ongoing.
5. Relevant data are documented in a retrievable form.

Standard II. Diagnosis

THE NURSE ANALYZES THE ASSESSMENT DATA IN DETER-MINING DIAGNOSES.

Measurement Criteria

1. Diagnoses are derived from the assessment data.
2. Diagnoses are validated with the client, significant others, and health care providers, when possible.
3. Diagnoses are documented in a manner that facilitates the determination of expected outcomes and plan of care.

Standard III. Outcome Identification

THE NURSE IDENTIFIES EXPECTED OUTCOMES INDIVIDUAL-
IZED TO THE CLIENT.

Measurement Criteria
1. Outcomes are derived from the diagnoses.
2. Outcomes are documented as measurable goals.
3. Outcomes are mutually formulated with the client and
   health care providers, when possible.
4. Outcomes are realistic in relation to the client's present and
   potential capabilities.
5. Outcomes are attainable in relation to resources available to
   the client.
6. Outcomes include a time estimate for attainment.
7. Outcomes provide direction for continuity of care.

Standard IV. Planning

THE NURSE DEVELOPS A PLAN OF CARE THAT PRESCRIBES
INTERVENTIONS TO ATTAIN EXPECTED OUTCOMES.

Measurement Criteria
1. The plan is individualized to the client's condition or needs.
2. The plan is developed with the client, significant others, and
   health care providers, when appropriate.
3. The plan reflects current nursing practice.
4. The plan is documented.
5. The plan provides for continuity of care.

Standard V. Implementation

THE NURSE IMPLEMENTS THE INTERVENTIONS IDENTIFIED IN THE PLAN OF CARE.

Measurement Criteria

1. Interventions are consistent with the established plan of care.
2. Interventions are implemented in a safe and appropriate manner.
3. Interventions are documented.

Standard VI. Evaluation

THE NURSE EVALUATES THE CLIENT'S PROGRESS TOWARD ATTAINMENT OF OUTCOMES.

Measurement Criteria

1. Evaluation is systematic and ongoing.
2. The client's responses to interventions are documented.
3. The effectiveness of interventions is evaluated in relation to outcomes.
4. Ongoing assessment data are used to revise diagnoses, outcomes, and the plan of care, as needed.
5. Revisions in diagnoses, outcomes, and the plan of care are documented.
6. The client, significant others, and health care providers are involved in the evaluation process, when appropriate.

STANDARDS OF PROFESSIONAL PERFORMANCE

Standard I. Quality of Care

THE NURSE SYSTEMATICALLY EVALUATES THE QUALITY AND EFFECTIVENESS OF NURSING PRACTICE.

Measurement Criteria

1. The nurse participates in quality of care activities as appropriate to the individual's position, education, and practice environment. Such activities may include:

   - Identification of aspects of care important for quality monitoring.
   - Identification of indicators used to monitor quality and effectiveness of nursing care.
   - Collection of data to monitor quality and effectiveness of nursing care.
   - Analysis of quality data to identify opportunities for improving care.
   - Formulation of recommendations to improve nursing practice or client outcomes.
   - Implementation of activities to enhance the quality of nursing practice.
   - Participation on interdisciplinary teams that evaluate clinical practice or health services.
   - Development of policies and procedures to improve quality of care.

2. The nurse uses the results of quality of care activities to initiate changes in practice.

3. The nurse uses the results of quality of care activities to initiate changes throughout the health care delivery system, as appropriate.

Standard II. Performance Appraisal

THE NURSE EVALUATES HIS/HER OWN NURSING PRACTICE IN RELATION TO PROFESSIONAL PRACTICE STANDARDS AND RELEVANT STATUTES AND REGULATIONS.

Measurement Criteria

1. The nurse engages in performance appraisal on a regular basis, identifying areas of strength as well as areas for professional/ practice development.
2. The nurse seeks constructive feedback regarding his/her own practice.
3. The nurse takes action to achieve goals identified during performance appraisal.
4. The nurse participates in peer review as appropriate.

Standard III. Education

THE NURSE ACQUIRES AND MAINTAINS CURRENT KNOWLEDGE IN NURSING PRACTICE.

Measurement Criteria

1. The nurse participates in ongoing educational activities related to clinical knowledge and professional issues.
2. The nurse seeks experiences to maintain clinical skills.
3. The nurse seeks knowledge and skills appropriate to the practice setting.

Standard IV. Collegiality

THE NURSE CONTRIBUTES TO THE PROFESSIONAL DEVEL-
OPMENT OF PEERS, COLLEAGUES, AND OTHERS.

Measurement Criteria

1. The nurse shares knowledge and skills with colleagues and others.
2. The nurse provides peers with constructive feedback regarding their practice.
3. The nurse contributes to an environment that is conducive to clinical education of nursing students, as appropriate.

Standard V. Ethics

THE NURSE'S DECISIONS AND ACTIONS ON BEHALF OF CLI-
ENTS ARE DETERMINED IN AN ETHICAL MANNER.

Measurement Criteria

1. The nurse's practice is guided by the *Code for Nurses.*[7]
2. The nurse maintains client confidentiality.
3. The nurse acts as a client advocate.
4. The nurse delivers care in a nonjudgmental and nondiscriminatory manner that is sensitive to client diversity.
5. The nurse delivers care in a manner that preserves/protects client autonomy, dignity, and rights.
6. The nurse seeks available resources to help formulate ethical decisions.

Standard VIII. Resource Utilization

THE NURSE CONSIDERS FACTORS RELATED TO SAFETY, EF-
FECTIVENESS, AND COST IN PLANNING AND DELIVERING
CLIENT CARE.

Measurement Criteria

> 1. The nurse evaluates factors related to safety, effectiveness, and cost when two or more practice options would result in the same expected client outcome.
>
> 2. The nurse assigns tasks or delegates care based on the needs of the client and the knowledge and skill of the provider selected.
>
> 3. The nurse assists the client and significant others in identifying and securing appropriate services available to address health-related needs.

GLOSSARY

CONTINUITY OF CARE. An interdisciplinary process that includes clients and significant others in the development of a coordinated plan of care. This process facilitates the client's transition between settings, based on changing needs and available resources.

CRITERIA. Relevant, measurable indicators of the standards of clinical nursing practice.

GUIDELINES. Describe a process of client care management which has the potential of improving the quality of clinical and consumer decision making. Guidelines are systematically developed statements based on available scientific evidence and expert opinion.

NURSING. The diagnosis and treatment of human responses to actual or potential health problems.[6]

STANDARD. Authoritative statement enunciated and promulgated by the profession by which the quality of practice, service, or education can be judged.

STANDARDS OF NURSING PRACTICE. Authoritative statements that describe a level of care or performance common to the profession of nursing by which the quality of nursing practice can be judged. Standards of clinical nursing practice include both standards of care and standards of professional performance.

STANDARDS OF CARE. Authoritative statements that describe a competent level of clinical nursing practice demonstrated through assessment, diagnosis, outcome identification, planning, implementation, and evaluation.

STANDARDS OF PROFESSIONAL PERFORMANCE. Authoritative statements that describe a competent level of behavior in the professional role, including activities related to quality of care, performance appraisal, education, collegiality, ethics, collaboration, research, and resource utilization.

REFERENCES

1. American Nurses Association. 1973. *Standards of Nursing Practice.* Washington, DC: American Nurses Association.

2. American Nurses Association. 1988. *Standards for Organized Nursing Services and Responsibilities of Nurse Administrators Across All Settings.* Washington, DC: American Nurses Association.

3. American Nurses Association. 1990. *Standards for Nursing Staff Development.* Washington, DC: American Nurses Association.

4. American Nurses Association. 1984. *Standards for Professional Nursing Education.* Washington, DC: American Nurses Association.

5. American Nurses Association. 1984. *Standards for Continuing Education in Nursing.* Washington, DC: American Nurses Association.

6. American Nurses Association. 1980. *Nursing: A Social Policy Statement.* Washington, DC: American Nurses Association.

7. American Nurses Association. 1985. *Code for Nurses with Interpretive Statements.* Washington, DC: American Nurses Association.

8. American Nurses Association. 1987. *The Scope of Nursing Practice.* Washington, DC: American Nurses Association.

9. American Nurses Association. 1989. *Education for Participation in Nursing Research.* Washington, DC: American Nurses Association.

APPENDIX E
Standards of Clinical Nursing Practice,
Second Edition (1998)

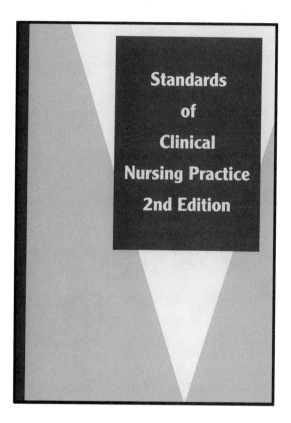

CONTENTS

PREFACE

Standards provide a means by which a profession clearly describes the focus of its activities, the recipients of service, and the responsibilities for which its practitioners are accountable. For professional nursing, the *Standards of Clinical Nursing Practice*[1] (the *Standards*) outlines the expectations of the full professional role within which all nurses must practice. The authority for the practice of nursing is based on a social contract that acknowledges professional rights and responsibilities as well as mechanisms for public accountability. The *Standards*, in conjunction with the definition of nursing practice, the statement of the scope of nursing practice, *Nursing's Social Policy Statement*,[2] and the *Code for Nurses with Interpretive Statements*,[3] contribute to a definitive description and understanding of nursing's accountability to the public.

The American Nurses Association (ANA) has actively engaged in standards development since the late 1960s. The first standards of practice for the nursing profession were published by ANA in 1973.[4] These standards were generic in nature and focused on the nursing process (assessment, diagnosis, planning, implementation, and evaluation). Over the years, specialty nursing organizations also developed standards of practice for nurses engaged in specialty practice such as critical care, perioperative, rehabilitation, psychiatric-mental health, and oncology nursing. Some of these standards were developed in collaboration with ANA; others were developed independently. Thus, the various sets of standards differed widely in purpose, scope, and format, and were limited in their ability to support an integrated nursing approach.

In 1990, a task force was charged by the ANA House of Delegates to define the nature and purpose of standards of practice for nursing. Included in their report was a recommendation that the 1973 *Standards of Nursing Practice* be revised. A participative process was instituted, incorporating broad input from state nurses associations and specialty nursing organizations. In 1991, the *Standards of Clinical Nursing Practice* was published by ANA after a long and fruitful collaboration with specialty nursing organizations. The *Standards* established a common language and consistent format to clarify and strengthen nursing's ability to articulate the scope of nursing practice in all clinical areas. What this process yielded was not only a set of professional clinical practice and performance standards for the profession, but also a framework within which specialty organizations and ANA could work together to develop standards and guidelines and foster a collaborative approach to decision-making.

Since that time, these standards have shaped nursing practice. They have helped nurses and other interested individuals and groups to understand what nursing encompasses and the activities for which nurses are accountable. Given the current health care environment, this has been particularly important as health care delivery and its financing have been radically transformed. The *Standards* document has increasingly been utilized to articulate what nursing is, what nurses do, and responsibilities for which nurses are accountable. The fact that the *Standards* reflects all of professional nursing has been especially beneficial. These are the standards by which all nurses practice. Specialty standards continue to be developed to reflect specific areas of nursing practice, yet the shared framework of the *Standards of Clinical Nursing Practice* unites the profession.

In 1995, the ANA Congress of Nursing Practice charged the Committee on Nursing Practice Standards and Guidelines with establishing a process for periodic review and revision, when necessary, of the *Standards of Clinical Nursing Practice*. This document is that product.

To accomplish this charge, the Committee instituted a process, incorporating wide input from state nurses associations, including individual members, and specialty nursing organizations. This joint collaboration had formed the basis of the development of the 1991 *Standards*. The process which was used in this review and revision incorporated three methods of data collection:

(1) an assessment of the congruency of the *Standards* with other ANA documents, e.g., *Nursing's Social Policy Statement*;

(2) a survey of individual nurses as to their perceptions of the frequency of use and relevancy of the *Standards* to their practice; and

(3) a survey of nursing organizations as to the usefulness of the *Standards* in regulatory and legislative activities.

From this process, extensive data regarding the *Standards* were obtained from nurses throughout the country. This information will be helpful in directing efforts toward the dissemination and utilization of the *Standards*.

Additional benefits have been achieved in this process. First, affirmation has been generated regarding the importance and usefulness of the *Standards*. In ways both written and oral, formal and informal, nurses have expressed support for the existence of the *Standards* and for its importance in shaping and collectively defining nursing practice.

Second, a collaborative process has been refined which can be used for subsequent evaluation and revision of the *Standards*. This process incorporates the feedback of individual nurses across the country, as well as members of the state nurses associations and specialty nursing organizations. Cycling every five years, the process will foster a thoughtful, timely, predictable review.

While much work has been done by hundreds of individuals with the revision and publication of the 1998 edition of the *Standards of Clinical Nursing Practice*, the real work begins now. Taking the written word and incorporating it meaningfully into practice settings across the country is now the task. Improving the health and well-being of all individuals through the significant and visible contributions of nurses utilizing standard-based practice must be the focus of the profession.

INTRODUCTION

Definition and Role of Standards

Standards are authoritative statements by which the nursing profession describes the responsibilities for which its practitioners are accountable. Consequently, standards reflect the values and priorities of the profession. Standards provide direction for professional nursing practice and a framework for the evaluation of practice. Written in measurable terms, standards also define the nursing profession's accountability to the public and the client outcomes for which nurses are responsible.

Development of Standards

Standards of professional nursing practice may pertain to general or specialty practice. A professional nursing organization has a responsibility to its membership and to the public it serves to develop standards of practice. As the professional organization for all registered nurses, ANA is responsible for developing generic standards that apply to the practice of all professional nurses. Standards do, however, belong to the profession and, thus, require broad input into their development and revision.

This publication sets forth standards of clinical nursing practice. It has been developed by ANA, in collaboration with numerous specialty nursing organizations and groups, for the nursing profession. The *Standards of Clinical Nursing Practice* describes a competent level of professional nursing care and professional performance common to all nurses engaged in clinical practice.

Assumptions

The *Standards of Clinical Nursing Practice* focuses primarily on the processes of providing nursing care and performing professional role activities. These standards apply to all nurses in all areas of clinical practice despite the tremendous variability in environments in which nurses practice. Recognizing the link between the professional work environment and the nurse's ability to deliver care, employers must provide an environment supportive of nursing practice.

A second assumption is that nursing care is individualized to meet a particular patient's unique needs and situation. This includes respect for the patient's and family's goals and preferences in developing and implementing a plan of care. Given that one of the nurse's primary responsibilities is patient education, nurses provide clients with appropriate information to make informed decisions regarding their health care and treatment, including health promotion, prevention of disease, and attainment of a peaceful death.

The third assumption is that the nurse establishes a partnership with the patient, family, and other health care providers. In this partnership, the nurse works collaboratively to coordinate the care provided to the patient. The degree of participation by the patient and family will vary based upon their preference and ability.

Organizing Principles of *Standards of Clinical Nursing Practice*

According to *Nursing's Social Policy Statement*, "the recipients of nursing care are individuals, groups, families, or communities. . . . The recipient(s) of nursing care can be referred to as patient(s), client(s), or person(s)."[2] The *Standards of Clinical Nursing Practice* uses the terms "patient" and "family" to indicate the person(s) to whom the nurse is providing services as sanctioned by the state nurse practice acts. Care can be provided to "assist the (patient), sick or well, in the performance of those activities contributing to health or its recovery (or to peaceful death) that (the patient) would perform unaided (if the patient had) the necessary strength, will, or knowledge. And to do this in such a way as to help (the patient) gain independence as rapidly as possible."[5] The cultural, racial, and ethnic diversity of the patient must always be taken into account in providing nursing services.

The *Standards of Clinical Nursing Practice* is generic in nature and applies to all registered nurses engaged in clinical practice, regardless of clinical specialty, practice setting, or educational preparation. Standards that further define the responsibilities of nurses engaged in specialty practice or nurses who function at advanced levels of clinical practice are determined by those nursing specialties and appropriate groups within ANA.

Professional nursing organizations and groups within ANA that represent nurses practicing in specialty areas will develop standards by building on the *Standards of Clinical Nursing Practice* and developing specific criteria for defining expectations associated with their particular area of clinical practice. Nurses practicing at an advanced level will be accountable for meeting the basic standards of clinical nursing practice, as well as the *Scope and Standards of Advanced Practice Registered Nursing*.[6]

The *Standards of Clinical Nursing Practice* consists of "Standards of Care" and "Standards of Professional Performance," which include the following:

Standards of Care
- Assessment
- Diagnosis
- Outcome Identification
- Planning
- Implementation
- Evaluation

Standards of Professional Performance
- Quality of Care
- Performance Appraisal
- Education
- Collegiality
- Ethics
- Collaboration
- Research
- Resource Utilization

Standards of Care

The six Standards of Care describe a competent level of nursing care as demonstrated by the nursing process, including assessment, diagnosis, outcome identification, planning, implementation, and evaluation. The nursing process encompasses all significant actions taken by nurses in providing care to all clients, and forms the foundation of clinical decision-making. Several themes cut across all areas of nursing practice and reflect nursing responsibilities for all patients. These themes provide an additional dimension for attention and include:

- providing age-appropriate and culturally and ethnically sensitive care
- maintaining a safe environment
- educating patients about healthy practices and treatment modalities
- assuring continuity of care
- coordinating the care across settings and among caregivers
- managing information
- communicating effectively

These themes will be reflected in the measurement criteria associated with various standards in the *Standards* document, although the wording may be different. They are highlighted here because they (1) are fundamental to many of the standards; and (2) have emerged as being consistently and significantly influential in nursing practice today. With the next revision of the *Standards,* some of these themes will undoubtedly evolve into standard statements in themselves.

Standards of Professional Performance

The eight Standards of Professional Performance describe a competent level of behavior in the professional role — including activities related to quality of care, performance appraisal, education, collegiality, ethics, collaboration, research, and resource utilization. All nurses are expected to engage in professional role activities appropriate to their education and position. Ultimately, nurses are accountable to themselves, their patients, and their peers for their professional actions.

Criteria

Criteria are key indicators of competent practice. The *Standards of Clinical Nursing Practice* includes criteria that allow the standards to be measured. For the standards to be met, all criteria must be met. Standards should remain stable over time, as they reflect the philosophical values of the profession. However, criteria can be revised to incorporate advancements in scientific knowledge and clinical practice. Criteria must remain consistent with current nursing practice and research.

Throughout this document, terms such as "appropriate," "pertinent," and "realistic" are used. A document like this one cannot account for all possible scenarios that the professional nurse might encounter in clinical practice. The nurse will need to exercise judgment based on education and experience in determining what is appropriate, pertinent, or realistic. Further direction may be available from documents such as guidelines for practice or agency standards, policies, procedures, and protocols.

Guidelines

Guidelines describe a process of patient care management which has the potential for improving the quality of clinical and consumer decision-making. As systematically developed statements based on available scientific evidence and expert opinion, guidelines address the care of specific patient populations or phenomena, whereas standards provide a broad framework for practice.

Summary

The *Standards of Clinical Nursing Practice* delineates the professional responsibilities of all registered nurses engaged in clinical practice, regardless of setting. The *Standards of Clinical Nursing Practice* and nursing practice guidelines could serve as a basis for:

- quality improvement systems
- data bases
- regulatory systems
- health care reimbursement and financing methodologies
- development and evaluation of nursing service delivery systems and organizational structures
- certification activities
- job descriptions and performance appraisals

- agency policies, procedures, and protocols
- educational offerings

In order to best serve the public health and the nursing profession, nursing must continue its efforts to develop standards of practice and practice guidelines. Nursing must examine how standards and practice guidelines can be disseminated and used most effectively to enhance and promote the quality of clinical practice. In addition, standards and practice guidelines must be evaluated on an ongoing basis, with revisions made as necessary. The dynamic nature of the health care environment and the growing body of nursing research provide both the impetus and the opportunity for nursing to ensure competent clinical practice and promote ongoing professional development and client care.

STANDARDS OF CARE

Standard I. Assessment

THE NURSE COLLECTS PATIENT HEALTH DATA.

Measurement Criteria

1. Data collection involves the patient, family, and other health care providers as appropriate.

2. The priority of data collection activities is determined by the patient's immediate condition or needs.

3. Pertinent data are collected using appropriate assessment techniques and instruments.

4. Relevant data are documented in a retrievable form.

5. The data collection process is systematic and ongoing.

Standard II. Diagnosis

THE NURSE ANALYZES THE ASSESSMENT DATA IN DETERMINING DIAGNOSES.

Measurement Criteria

1. Diagnoses are derived from the assessment data.

2. Diagnoses are validated with the patient, family, and other health care providers, when possible and appropriate.

3. Diagnoses are documented in a manner that facilitates the determination of expected outcomes and plan of care.

Standard III. Outcome Identification

THE NURSE IDENTIFIES EXPECTED OUTCOMES INDIVIDU-ALIZED TO THE PATIENT.

Measurement Criteria

1. Outcomes are derived from the diagnoses.

2. Outcomes are mutually formulated with the patient, family, and other health care providers, when possible and appropriate.

3. Outcomes are culturally appropriate and realistic in relation to the patient's present and potential capabilities.

4. Outcomes are attainable in relation to resources available to the patient.

5. Outcomes include a time estimate for attainment.

6. Outcomes provide direction for continuity of care.

7. Outcomes are documented as measurable goals.

Standard IV. Planning

THE NURSE DEVELOPS A PLAN OF CARE THAT PRESCRIBES INTERVENTIONS TO ATTAIN EXPECTED OUTCOMES.

Measurement Criteria

1. The plan is individualized to the patient (e.g., age-appropriate, culturally sensitive) and the patient's condition or needs.

2. The plan is developed with the patient, family, and other health care providers, as appropriate.

3. The plan reflects current nursing practice.

4. The plan provides for continuity of care.

5. Priorities for care are established.

6. The plan is documented.

Standard V. Implementation

THE NURSE IMPLEMENTS THE INTERVENTIONS IDENTIFIED IN THE PLAN OF CARE.

Measurement Criteria

1. Interventions are consistent with the established plan of care.

2. Interventions are implemented in a safe, timely, and appropriate manner.

3. Interventions are documented.

Standard VI. Evaluation

THE NURSE EVALUATES THE PATIENT'S PROGRESS TOWARD ATTAINMENT OF OUTCOMES.

Measurement Criteria

1. Evaluation is systematic, ongoing, and criterion-based.

2. The patient, family, and other health care providers are involved in the evaluation process, as appropriate.

3. Ongoing assessment data are used to revise diagnoses, outcomes, and the plan of care, as needed.

Nursing: Scope and Standards of Practice

4. Revisions in diagnoses, outcomes, and the plan of care are documented.

5. The effectiveness of interventions is evaluated in relation to outcomes.

6. The patient's responses to interventions are documented.

STANDARDS OF PROFESSIONAL PERFORMANCE

Standard I. Quality of Care

THE NURSE SYSTEMATICALLY EVALUATES THE QUALITY AND EFFECTIVENESS OF NURSING PRACTICE.

Measurement Criteria

1. The nurse participates in quality of care activities as appropriate to the nurse's education and position. Such activities may include:
   - identification of aspects of care important for quality monitoring
   - analysis of quality data to identify opportunities for improving care
   - development of policies, procedures, and practice guidelines to improve quality of care
   - identification of indicators used to monitor quality and effectiveness of nursing care
   - collection of data to monitor quality and effectiveness of nursing care
   - formulation of recommendations to improve nursing practice or patient outcomes
   - implementation of activities to enhance the quality of nursing practice
   - participation on interdisciplinary teams that evaluate clinical practice or health services

2. The nurse uses the results of quality of care activities to initiate changes in nursing practice.

3. The nurse uses the results of quality of care activities to initiate changes throughout the health care delivery system, as appropriate.

Nursing: Scope and Standards of Practice

Standard II. Performance Appraisal

THE NURSE EVALUATES ONE'S OWN NURSING PRACTICE IN RELATION TO PROFESSIONAL PRACTICE STANDARDS AND RELEVANT STATUTES AND REGULATIONS.

Measurement Criteria

1. The nurse engages in performance appraisal on a regular basis, identifying areas of strength as well as areas where professional development would be beneficial.

2. The nurse seeks constructive feedback regarding one's own practice.

3. The nurse takes action to achieve goals identified during performance appraisal.

4. The nurse participates in peer review as appropriate.

5. The nurse's practice reflects knowledge of current professional practice standards, laws, and regulations.

Standard III. Education

THE NURSE ACQUIRES AND MAINTAINS CURRENT KNOWLEDGE AND COMPETENCY IN NURSING PRACTICE.

Measurement Criteria

1. The nurse participates in ongoing educational activities related to clinical knowledge and professional issues.

2. The nurse seeks experiences that reflect current clinical practice in order to maintain current clinical skills and competence.

3. The nurse acquires knowledge and skills appropriate to the specialty area and practice setting.

Standard IV. Collegiality

THE NURSE INTERACTS WITH, AND CONTRIBUTES TO THE PROFESSIONAL DEVELOPMENT OF, PEERS AND OTHER HEALTH CARE PROVIDERS AS COLLEAGUES.

Measurement Criteria

1. The nurse shares knowledge and skills with colleagues.

2. The nurse provides peers with constructive feedback regarding their practice.

3. The nurse interacts with colleagues to enhance one's own professional nursing practice.

4. The nurse contributes to an environment that is conducive to the clinical education of nursing students, other health care students, and other employees, as appropriate.

5. The nurse contributes to a supportive and healthy work environment.

Standard V. Ethics

THE NURSE'S DECISIONS AND ACTIONS ON BEHALF OF PATIENTS ARE DETERMINED IN AN ETHICAL MANNER.

Measurement Criteria

1. The nurse's practice is guided by the *Code for Nurses*.[3]

2. The nurse maintains patient confidentiality within legal and regulatory parameters.

3. The nurse acts as a patient advocate and assists patients in developing skills so they can advocate for themselves.

4. The nurse delivers care in a nonjudgmental and nondiscriminatory manner that is sensitive to patient diversity.

5. The nurse delivers care in a manner that preserves patient autonomy, dignity, and rights.

6. The nurse seeks available resources in formulating ethical decisions.

Standard VI. Collaboration

THE NURSE COLLABORATES WITH THE PATIENT, FAMILY, AND OTHER HEALTH CARE PROVIDERS IN PROVIDING PATIENT CARE.

Measurement Criteria

1. The nurse communicates with the patient, family, and other health care providers regarding patient care and nursing's role in the provision of care.

2. The nurse collaborates with the patient, family, and other health care providers in the formulation of overall goals and the plan of care, and in decisions related to care and the delivery of services.

3. The nurse consults with other health care providers for patient care, as needed.

4. The nurse makes referrals, including provisions for continuity of care, as needed.

Standard VII. Research

THE NURSE USES RESEARCH FINDINGS IN PRACTICE.

Measurement Criteria

1. The nurse utilizes best available evidence, preferably research data, to develop the plan of care and interventions.

2. The nurse participates in research activities as appropriate to the nurse's education and position. Such activities may include:
   - identifying clinical problems suitable for nursing research
   - participating in data collection
   - participating in a unit, organization, or community research committee or program
   - sharing research activities with others
   - conducting research
   - critiquing research for application to practice
   - using research findings in the development of policies, procedures, and practice guidelines for patient care

Standard VIII. Resource Utilization

THE NURSE CONSIDERS FACTORS RELATED TO SAFETY, EFFECTIVENESS, AND COST IN PLANNING AND DELIVERING PATIENT CARE.

Measurement Criteria

1. The nurse evaluates factors related to safety, effectiveness, availability, and cost when choosing between two or more practice options that would result in the same expected patient outcome.

2. The nurse assists the patient and family in identifying and

securing appropriate and available services to address health-related needs.

3. The nurse assigns or delegates tasks as defined by the state nurse practice acts and according to the knowledge and skills of the designated caregiver.

4. If the nurse assigns or delegates tasks, it is based on the needs and condition of the patient, the potential for harm, the stability of the patient's condition, the complexity of the task, and the predictability of the outcome.

5. The nurse assists the patient and family in becoming informed consumers about the cost, risks, and benefits of treatment and care.

KEY TERMS

Assessment—A systematic, dynamic process by which the nurse, through interaction with the client, significant others, and health care providers, collects and analyzes data about the client. Data may include the following dimensions: physical, psychological, sociocultural, spiritual, cognitive, functional abilities, developmental, economic, and life-style.

Continuity of Care—An interdisciplinary process that includes clients and significant others in the development of a coordinated plan of care. This process facilitates the client's transition between settings, based on changing needs and available resources.

Criteria—Relevant, measurable indicators of the standards of clinical nursing practice.

Diagnosis—A clinical judgment about the client's response to actual or potential health conditions or needs. The diagnosis provides the basis for determination of a plan of care to achieve expected outcomes.

Evaluation—The process of determining both the client's progress toward the attainment of expected outcomes and the effectiveness of nursing care.

Family—Family of origin or significant others as identified by the patient.

Guidelines—Describe a process of client care management which has the potential of improving the quality of clinical and consumer decision-making. Guidelines are systematically developed statements based on available scientific evidence and expert opinion.

Health Care Providers—Individuals with special expertise who provide health care services or assistance to clients. They may include nurses, physicians, psychologists, social workers, nutritionists/dieticians, and various therapists.

Implementation—May include any or all of these activities: intervening, delegating, coordinating. The client, significant others, or health care providers may be designated to implement interventions within the plan of care.

Nurse—An individual who is licensed by a state agency to practice as a registered nurse.

Nursing—The diagnosis and treatment of human responses to actual or potential health problems.[6]

Outcomes—Measurable, expected, patient-focused goals that translate into observable behaviors.

Patient—Recipient of nursing care. The term patient is used in the *Standards* to provide consistency and brevity, bearing in mind that the terms *client* or *individual* might be better choices in some instances. When the patient is an individual client, the focus is on the health state, problems, or needs of a single person. When the patient is a family or group, the focus is on the health state of the unit as a whole or the reciprocal effects of an individual's health state on the other members of the unit. When the patient is a community, the focus is on personal and environmental health and the health risks of population groups.

Plan of Care—Comprehensive outline of care to be delivered to attain expected outcomes.

Quality of Care—Quality of care is the degree to which health services for individuals and populations increase the likelihood of desired health outcomes and are consistent with current professional knowledge.

Recipients of Nursing Care—Patients, groups, families, communities, or populations.

Standard—Authoritative statement enunciated and promulgated by the profession by which the quality of practice, service, or education can be judged.

Standards of Care—Authoritative statements that describe a competent level of clinical nursing practice demonstrated through assessment, diagnosis, outcome identification, planning, implementation, and evaluation.

Standards of Nursing Practice—Authoritative statements that describe a level of care or performance common to the profession of nursing by which the quality of nursing practice can be judged. Standards of clinical nursing practice include both standards of care and standards of professional performance.

Standards of Professional Performance—Authoritative statements that describe a competent level of behavior in the professional role, including activities related to quality of care, performance appraisal, education, collegiality, ethics, collaboration, research, and resource utilization.

REFERENCES

1. American Nurses Association. 1991. *Standards of Clinical Nursing Practice.* Washington, DC: American Nurses Association.

2. American Nurses Association. 1995. *Nursing's Social Policy Statement.* Washington, DC: American Nurses Association.

3. American Nurses Association. 1985. *Code for Nurses with Interpretive Statements.* Washington, DC: American Nurses Association.

4. American Nurses Association. 1973. *Standards of Nursing Practice.* Washington, DC: American Nurses Association.

5. Henderson, V. 1997. *Basic Principles of Nursing Care*, p. 22. Geneva: International Council of Nurses. Reprinted with permission.

6. American Nurses Association. 1996. *Scope and Standards of Advanced Practice Registered Nursing.* Washington, DC: American Nurses Association.

Nursing: Scope and Standards of Practice

INDEX

Note: Entries designated with a calendar year in brackets indicates an entry from an earlier edition or predecessor publication. [1987] is *The Scope of Nursing Practice.* [1973] is *Standards of Nursing Practice.* [1991] is *Standards of Clinical Nursing Practice.* [1998] is *Standards of Clinical Nursing Practice, 2nd Edition.*

C

Care recipient. *See* Patient

Care standards. *See* Standards
of practice

Caregiver (defined), 47

Case management. *See* Coordination
of care

Certification and credentialing
leadership and, 44
nursing and, 11, 12, 13, 20
quality of practice and, 34
standards and, 6
[1987], 69–70

Certified Nurse Midwife, 8, 14, 15
[1991], 78

Certified Registered Nurse
Anesthetist, 8, 14–15
[1991], 78

Client. *See* Patient

Clinical Nurse Specialist
(CNS), 8, 14, 15
[1991], 78

*Code of Ethics for Nurses with
Interpretive Statements*, 9, 11, 18, 39
intended use, *vii*
review process, *viii*
[1991], 89
[1998], 95, 110
See also Ethics

Collaboration, 11
implementation and, 26
standard of professional
performance, 38
[1998], 111
See also Interdisciplinary health
care teams

Collegiality
diagnosis and, 22
standard of professional
performance, 37
[1991], 89
[1998], 110

Communication
collaboration and, 38
collegiality and, 37
consultation and, 29
evaluation and, 31
leadership and, 45
research and, 41

Community health care, 26
See also Practice settings

Competence assessment. *See*
Certification and credentialing

Confidentiality, 39
[1991], 89
[1998], 111

Consultation, 10, 17
collaboration and, 38
research and, 41
standard of practice, 29

Continuing education. *See*
Professional Development

Continuity of care
collaboration and, 38
[1998], 111
defined, 47
[1991], 91
[1998], 114
outcome identification and, 23
[1991], 85
[1998], 105
planning and, 24
[1991], 85
[1998], 106

Coordination of care
leadership and, 44
standard of practice, 27
See also Interdisciplinary
healthcare teams

Cost control, 11, 18
outcome identification and, 23
planning and, 24
prescriptive authority and, 30
quality of practice and, 33

resource utilization and, 42, 43
    [1991], 90
    [1998], 112
    standards and, 6
Cost-effectiveness. *See* Cost control
Council on Certification of Nurse
    Anesthetists, 15
Credentialing. *See* Certification and
    credentialing
Criteria, 4
    assessment, 21
    collaboration, 38
    collegiality, 37
    consultation, 29
    coordination of care, 27
    defined, 5, 47
        [1991], 91
        [1998], 114
    diagnosis, 22
    education, 35
    ethics, 39
    evaluation, 31–32
    health teaching and health
    promotion, 28
    implementation, 26–30
    leadership, 44–45
    outcome identification, 23
    planning, 24–25
    prescriptive authority and
    treatment, 30
    professional practice
    evaluation, 36
    quality of practice, 33–34
    research, 40–41
    resource utilization, 42–43
    [1973], 57–61
    [1991], 79–80, 84–90
    [1998],101–102, 104–113
Critical thinking, analysis, and
    synthesis, vii, 10, 11–12, 20
    assessment and, 21
    consultation and, 29

coordination of care and, 27
diagnosis and, 22
evaluation and, 31, 32
health promotion and, 28
planning and, 24
quality of practice and, 33
    [1991], 87
    [1998], 108
research and, 40, 41
Cultural competence, 10
    ethics and, [1991], 89
    health promotion and, 28
    organizing principle of nursing
        practice, 2
    outcome identification and, 23
        [1998], 105
    planning and, 24
        [1998], 105
    practice evaluation and, 36

D
Data (defined), 47
Data collection, 18
    assessment and, 21
        [1973], 58–59
        [1991], 84
        [1998], 104
    implementation, 26–30
    quality of practice and, 33
        [1991], 87
    research and, 40
        [1998], 112
    standards and, 6
Decision-making
    consultation and, 29
    guidelines and, 5
    leadership and, 45
    planning and, 25
    standards and, 12
    work environment and, 2
Delivery systems. *See* Nursing care
    delivery systems

Disease (defined), 47
Diagnosis
    assessment and, 21
    defined, 47
        [1991], 82
        [1998], 114
    evaluation and, 31
        [1991], 86
    implementation and, 26
    outcome identification and, 23
        [1998], 105
    planning and, 24
    standard of practice, 22
        [1973], 59
        [1991], 84
        [1998], 104
Documentation
    assessment and, 21
        [1991], 84
        [1998], 104
    collaboration and, 38
    coordination of care and, 27
    diagnosis and, 22
        [1991], 84
        ]1998], 104
    education and, 35
    evaluation and, 31
        [1998], 107
    implementation and, 26
        [1991], 86
    outcome identification and, 23
        [1991], 84
        [1998], 105
    planning and, 24
        [1991], 85
        [1998], 106
    quality of practice and, 33

E
Economic issues. See Cost control
Education of nurses
    collaboration and, 38

collegiality and, 37
    [1991], 89
history, 7–9
importance of, 2, 16, 18, 19, 20
paths for registered nurses, 13–14
professional development and,
    10–11
research and, 40
standard of professional
    performance, 35
    [1991], 88
    [1998], 109–110
standards and, 6
    [1987] 66–67, 71–72
Education of patients and families.
    See Health teaching and health
    promotion
*Educational Preparation for Nurse
Practitioners and Assistants to
Nurses*, [1987], 71
Environment (defined), 47
Ethics
    code, *vii, viii,* 9, 11, 18, 39, 47
    outcome identification and, 23
    quality of practice and, 33
    research and, 19
    standard of professional
        performance, 39
        [1991], 89
        [1998], 110
Evaluation
    defined, 47
        [1991], 82
        [1998], 114
    standard of practice, 31–32
        [1973], 61
        [1991], 86
        [1998], 106–107
Evidence-based practice, 12, 17
    assessment and, 21
    consultation and, 29
    defined, 48

implementation and, 26
leadership and, 45
origins, 7
outcome identification and, 23
planning and, 24
prescriptive authority and, 30
See also Research
Expected outcomes (defined), 47
See also Outcomes

F
Family
assessment and, 21
collaboration and, 38
defined, 48
[1998], 114
diagnosis and, 22
evaluation and, 31, 32
outcome identification and, 23
planning and, 24
relationship with nurse, 2
respect for, 2
resource utilization and, 42
Financial issues. *See* Cost control

G
Guidelines
defined, 5, 48
[1991], 76
[1998], 102, 114
outcome identification and, 23
standards and, 5, 6

H
Health (defined), 48
Health teaching and health promotion
ethics and, 39
planning and, 24
resource utilization and, 42
standard of practice, 28
[1973], 60–61

Healthcare policy
evaluation and, 31, 32
leadership and, 45
nursing and, 8–9, 20
quality of practice and, 33
[1991], 87
[1998], 108
research and, 40
[1998], 112
standards and, 6
Healthcare providers
assessment and, 21
collaboration and, 38
[1998], 111
defined, 48
[1991], 83
[1998], 114
diagnosis and, 22
evaluation and, 31
[1998], 106
outcome identification and, 23
[1998], 105
partnership with nursing, 2
[1991], 80–81
planning and, 24
See also Interdisciplinary
healthcare teams
Holism in nursing, 10, 12
defined, 48
Human resources
leadership and, 44
shortage of nurses, 19
standards and, 6
See also Professional development

I
Illness (defined), 48
Implementation
coordination of care and, 27
defined, 48
[1991], 82
[1998], 115

evaluation and, 31
planning and, 24
standard of practice, 26–30
[1991], 86
[1998], 106
Information, 2, 4, 19, 21, 27–30, 38, 45
defined, 48
See also Data collection and usage
Interdisciplinary healthcare teams,
10, 11
collaboration and, 38
collegiality and, 37
coordination of care and, 27
defined, 48
ethics and, 39
implementation and, 26
leadership and, 45
planning and, 25
quality of practice and, 33
[1991], 87
[1998], 108
resource utilization and, 42
See also Collaboration
Interventions
implementation and, 26
[1991], 86
[1998], 106
planning and, 24
research and, 7

K
Knowledge
defined, 48
[1987], 66–67
See also Information

L
Laws, statutes, and regulations
ethics and, 39
evaluation and, 31
planning and, 24
practice evaluation and, 36
[1998], 109

private nursing practice and, 8
standards and, 6
[1987], 68–70
See also Ethics
Leadership
coordination of care and, 27
standard of professional
performance, 44–45
Legal issues. See Laws, statutes, and
regulations
Licensing. See Certification and
credentialing

M
Measurement criteria. See Criteria
Medicaid and Medicare, 9
Mentoring, 20
collegiality and, 37
leadership and, 44
Midwifery. See Certified Nurse
Midwife
Models of nursing, 8
Multidisciplinary healthcare, 11, 15
(defined), 48
See also Interdisciplinary
healthcare teams

N
National Center for Nursing
Research, 7–8
National Council of State Boards of
Nursing, [1987], 71–72
National Federation of Licensed
Practical Nurses, [1987], 71
National Institutes of Health, 8
National Sample Survey of
Registered Nurses (NSSRN), 9
Nightingale, Florence, 7, 54
Nurse Practitioner, 8, 14, 16
[1991], 78
Nursing
armed forces and, 8
defined, *vii*, 7

Nursing: Scope and Standards of Practice

Nursing: Scope and Standards of Practice

Nursing: Scope and Standards of Practice